BLAGRAVE'S
Astrological Practice
OF
PHYSICK

DISCOVERING,
The true way to Cure all Kinds of Diseases and Infirmities which are Naturally incident to the body of man.

BEING

Performed by such Herbs and Plants which grow within our own Nation, directing the way to Distil and Extract their Virtues and making up of Medicines.

ALSO,

A Discovery of some notable *Phylosophical Secrets* worthy of our knowledge, relating to a discovery of all kinds of *Evils*, whether Natural, or such which come from *Sorcery* or *Witchcraft*, or by being possessed of an Evil Spirit : directing how to call forth the said Evil Spirit out of any one which is possessed with sundry Examples thereof.

By *Joseph Blagrave* of *Reading* Gent. Student
In *Astrology* and *Physick*

London, Printed by S.G. and B.G. for *Obad. Blagrave* at the *Printing Press* in *Little Brittain*, 1671

Publisher's disclaimer: This is a book of herbalism and astrological medicine. It is not intended for lay readers, and the publisher is not responsible for the misuse of its contents. Also note that while I have made every effort to produce an accurate and exact copy of Blagrave's book and all the many ingredients in it, due to the poor condition of the original (a photocopy), along with the original's erratic spelling, combined with many obscurities, *the accuracy of the formulas in this book is not guaranteed. Proceed with caution, and at your own risk.*

On the cover: The city of Mainz, from Medieval Woodcut Illustrations, by Carol Belanger Grafton, published by Dover Publications, 1999; and, a Celtic border, from Celtic Frames and Borders, Dover Publications, 2000.

ISBN 978 1 933303 28 4

Copyright © 2010 by William R. Roell
All rights reserved

Published by
Astrology Classics

the publication division of
The Astrology Center of America
207 Victory Lane, Bel Air MD 21014

on line at www.AstroAmerica.com

Editor's Preface

Having seen the limited use that others have made of this book, I will use the Preface to explain some of its less-well understood terms.

<u>Plants and herbs</u>:
Blagrave starts with the usual list of plants and herbs, as ruled by the various planets. You will find much the same in Culpeper's Herbal, or, for that matter, in the Botanical Interlude in J. Lee Lehman's Essential Dignities (Whitford, 1989). Note that Blagrave's list, on pgs. 1 - 6, is not a complete catalogue of his ingredients, as a study of the recipes given on pgs. 83 - 109 will show. (Most of these can be found, alphabetized, in the first Appendix.)

<u>Perpetual almanac of planetary hours</u>:
The author gives a detailed, perpetual almanac of precise dates and times to gather the herbs ruled by the various planets. Which, in simple terms, is the first hour after sunrise on the appropriate day: Solar plants are to be harvested at sunrise on Sunday, Lunar planets at sunrise on Monday, Martian plants at sunrise on Tuesday, etc.

Regrettably, the dates that Blagrave gives, and which I have copies, are no longer valid, as he has given them in the Julian Calendar (also known as Old Style, or O.S.). To convert Blagrave's dates to the current Gregorian Calendar (also known as New Style, or N.S.), add ten days. January 1, to Blagrave, is January 11 to us.

Once the dates are converted, the times that Blagrave gives are valid if you are within a degree or two of the same latitude, north of the equator, as Reading, England (51° N 28"). In Europe, such places include London, Antwerp, Berlin, Warsaw, Brussels, Rotterdam and Leipzig.

A useful shortcut: Harvesting that occurs within the first half hour after sunrise will meet Blagrave's requirements, and this is regardless of latitude, longitude, time in use or the season of the year, presuming you have at least six hours between sunrise and sunset.

For those in need of precisely calculated planetary hours, the procedure, for daylight hours, is as follows:

Take the time of sunset. Convert to a 24 hour clock (in other words, sunset at 6:00 pm is 18:00). From this, subtract the time of sunrise.

Take the result, in hours and minutes, and convert to minutes.

Divide by 12. This is the length, in minutes, of one planetary hour. Add this interval to sunrise to get the first hour of the day. Add it again to get the second hour, a third time to get the third, etc. For Blagrave's purposes, the first and the eighth hours of the day are of importance. This sequence of hours ends at sunset.

Blagrave does not use nighttime hours, but if they are needed, they are calculated in the same manner as daytime hours:

Convert the time of sunset to the 24 hour clock, as before. Take the time of the next morning's sunrise and add 24 hours to it (this will make subtraction easier).

Subtract sunset from sunrise. Convert to minutes. Divide by 12. The result is the length of each nighttime hour. Add to sunset to get the first hour of night, add again to get the second nighttime hour, add a third time to get the third, etc. Similar to the daytime hours, this sequence ends at sunrise, when daytime hours again begin.

As Blagrave indicates in his tables, the difference in times, from one day to the next, are slight. The calculations show that daytime hours are longest in summer and shortest in winter, while nighttime hours are the reverse.

The order of rulerships of the hours are as follows: Saturn, Jupiter, Mars, Sun, Venus, Mercury, Moon. After which the series starts over again with Saturn. As Saturn rules the first hour after sunrise on Saturday, this sequence will make the 25th hour (the first hour of the next day, which is Sunday) to be ruled by the Sun.

Which is correct for the first hour of Sunday.

The rulers of the days of the week are as follows:
Sunday ruled by the Sun.
Monday ruled by the Moon.
Tuesday ruled by Mars.
Wednesday ruled by Mercury.
Thursday ruled by Jupiter.
Friday ruled by Venus.
Saturday ruled by Saturn.

Vary the ascendant:

Blagrave's insistence on precise dates and times of harvest are because he works in what I might call near-magic, where "magic" is defined as a world with more precise definitions. You might think of it as the difference between, say, a 1950 television set, and the latest high-definition TV set. While the two units are basically the same (they display pictures), the high-definition set works to much higher standards, and therefore gives much better results. So it is with magic, and so it is with Blagrave's cures.

Blagrave is saying that we can better heal the sick, can avoid death, can prolong life, if our medicine is more precise. More precise, more powerful. Herbs and plants, harvested at the precise time on the appropriate days, become super plants and herbs.

But to properly use these Super Herbs, we must have a superior understanding of the ailment in question. Otherwise our treatment is wasted, or is actually harmful. And here Blagrave makes a critical innovation with the decumbiture chart.

Ordinarily the decumbiture chart is set for the moment the patient takes to his bed, or, anymore, the moment the ambulance arrives. Failing that, the decumbiture is set for the time the astrological doctor is alerted to the situation. From the decumbiture alone, astrologers make the diagnosis.

Blagrave changes this in one critical respect. Blagrave insists the ascendant of the decumbiture match the appearance of the patient. He is, in fact, changing the time of the decumbiture on a wholesale basis. He fudges this by saying, well, you know, clocks can be wrong and we have to adjust the time accordingly. But he repeatedly says the decumbiture must be adjusted to resemble the patient.

This is a departure from all astrological rules, which insist on strict, even merciless, timekeeping. Nor is this ascendant to be made to match the patient's sun sign, moon sign, or ascendant, as few of Blagrave's patients would have known their birth dates.

The net result of these two innovations, (precisely harvested herbs, charts timed for appearance) is made clear in Blagrave's delineations of Moon in aspect with Mars or Saturn, when we compare Blagrave's definitions, with those given by William Lilly in Christian Astrology. As an example, here is Lilly's delineation of the Moon conjunct, square, or opposed to Mars in Virgo:

> Usually an alteration or flux in the Belly, or miseraicks follows this unlucky position, small Fevers, the original choler and melancholy, the Pulse remiss, eversion of the ventricle, loathing of food; death within thirty days, if the fortunes assist not.
>
> I have by experience found, the afflicted upon this aspect or aspects, to be tormented with the wind, cholic, many times weakness in the legs or near the ankles. Yet I never did find any Disease easily removable, if the Moon at the time of the decumbiture, or first falling ill, was afflicted by Mars in Virgo. (Christian Astrology, Book 2, pg. 279)

Here is the same delineation, Moon to Mars in Virgo, in Blagrave:

> Those who take their bed under this configuration, shall be subject to a Flux in the belly, small Fevers, the Pulse remiss, aversion of the Ventricle, also tormented with wind in the Belly or Guts, and Cholic, bad stomach many times, weakness or pains in the legs near the ankles ; the cause from original choler, melancholy, and sharp fretting humours. (pg. 64)

In surveying Lilly's delineations in Christian Astrology (Moon/Saturn, Moon/Mars, pgs. 273 - 282), Lilly forecasts death, directly or indirectly, in eight of the 24 possibilities (five under Saturn, three

Editor's Preface: Blagrave, Lilly, external healing vii

under Mars). Blagrave forecasts death not once, and not, as we might imagine, because he has already written the patient off, based on the decumbiture, for if it were as simple as that, he would say so. Blagrave's medicine is better. So let's have a look at it.

External healing, part 1: External healing assistance:
Modern medicine relies almost entirely on drugs. Traditional medicine was more colorful. Traditional techniques included teas (diet-drinks, to Blagrave), gruel, syrups, things to lick, cataplasms administered directly to the skin, ointments, fumes, bloodletting, suppositories, baths, bracelets, necklaces and more. With his super herbs and superior diagnosis, Blagrave is a master of all of these.

In particular, in many places in this book Blagrave exhorts the patient to wear three solar herbs in a small bag placed around the neck. From what he writes, Blagrave laments that this was not understood in his own day, and, regrettably, it is still not understood in ours. This is a pity.

Why solar herbs, and why around the neck? The answer, it turns out, is straightforward:

Anything "worn around the neck" is by definition not a choker, but a necklace. Necklaces commonly come to rest on the sternum, or breastbone. Which is directly next to the heart. The heart, as all astrologers know, is ruled by Leo, which, in its turn, is ruled by the Sun. Blagrave's use of a bag of solar herbs around the neck is his way of strengthening the heart itself. A weak heart, in fact, is the root cause of many illnesses and discomforts. Strengthen the heart, and half the work of healing is already done.

I myself suffer from a weak heart, for which I see a Chinese herbalist twice a month. Midway through this book, I realized what Blagrave was up to and became envious. But, alas, I am not an herbalist and no one I know has herbs harvested at the proper hours. I was in despair, but then remembered an old wedding ring, from a failed relationship. It was a man's, it was heavy, it was 18K gold. One Sunday at sunrise, I put it outside in the sun in a clear glass of salted water. A week later at sunrise I brought it indoors, tied it to a shoelace, and put it around my neck. My doctor was at first skeptical, but, six months later, my heartbeat has steadied, palpitations, which had been controlled with the doctor's "diet-drinks" are, with the addition of the ring, now virtually gone. For her part, the doctor is most curious.

The ring I wear weighs about .6 ounce. It has about .4 ounce of gold in it. I weigh about 200 pounds. I doubt the small gold crosses that many wear have enough gold in them to be of much use. A one-half ounce gold coin, worn about the neck, should do very well. It would be a much better use of the coin than merely letting it sit about in a vault or drawer.

Because what happens when we put herbs, or gold rings (or gold crosses) around our necks is that their radiance, or aura, or essence, or virtue (call it what you will) interacts with the essence, or aura, or radiance, or virtue (again, what you will) of the part of the body it is placed next to. Many people know the major organs of the body correspond to energy vortices, known as chakras, but few have any idea what to do with that knowledge. Blagrave gives us a useful introduction. When a substance that is friendly to a given chakra is placed next to it, the chakra is strengthened. When something not-so-friendly is placed next to a chakra, it is weakened.

This can be demonstrated by a simple experiment. It requires two people, one as subject, one as experimenter.

The subject makes a fist of the left hand, and places it directly over his heart. The right arm he extends straight out from his body. The experimenter, using both his arms, tries to push down the subject's right arm, the subject resisting as best he can. This establishes a base line, for future reference.

The subject now grasps a variety of small objects in his left hand, one at a time. He holds them next to his heart, whereupon the experimenter tries to push his right arm down, as before. Among the various items that can be tried in this way are vitamins, minerals, over the counter remedies (aspirin), prescription drugs, small fruits and vegetables, jewelry, stones (quartz), soap, alcohol, coins, small keepsakes and souvenirs, etc. An observer will see great variations in the strength of the subject.

This works for the same reason that Blagrave's three herbs in a bag around the neck work: Objects have auras, the body has its own aura, when the two are brought into contact, a reaction occurs. And it's not only with necklaces. This also includes copper bracelets (used for arthritis), ointments, creams, salves, cataplasms (plasters)

Editor's Preface: External healing

and much more. It is the true reason why we wear precious metals and stones as jewelry. They're not just ornamentation.

Blagrave exploits this more than you think. In addition to three herbs worn around the neck, he often advises hot cataplasms laid on the wrists. Why the wrists, and why hot? It helps to know a bit more about the body's energy field.

Because of what the hands do, they are energy openings into the body. The hands are how we contact the physical world around us. This world contains many energies, some of which are helpful, but many which are not. The body needs a way to both sense them, as well as keep them out.

For sensing, the body uses the minor chakras in the center of the palms themselves. Christians know this pair as the nail marks in the palms of the risen Christ. The marks were not due to the nails, but are in fact the man's palm chakras. (The nails were driven through the wrists, as the bones there will hold weight. The palms will not. Gruesome, but true.)

For its own safety, the body cuts off this sensing ability at the wrists, most likely through sheer bone mass. As a result of the blockage, the body is forced to route blood and nerves just under the skin. Blagrave exploits this entry point with carefully selected herbs, laid on hot, as cataplasms, to swell the blood vessels, enabling the body to take on more of the herbal energies. The reader will note that Blagrave does not use any of the other blood vessels near the skin, such as the jugular.

The jugular, uniquely, is used in jewelry, specifically earrings. Those who wear earrings change them from time to time. A clairvoyant once told me this was because the energies generated by jewels and precious metals in earrings interact directly with the blood streaming into the head. This interaction is two-way, for when the head that wears them generates powerful emotions, those emotions can be channeled by the precious metals and come to rest in the gems themselves, slowly polluting them. Over time this results in dissatisfaction with the item, resulting in its abandonment. Putting the items in strong salted water and placing them in strong sunlight for a week or two, will, in many cases, cleanse the jewels and restore the owner's interest in them. Which indicates the healing possibilities inherent in earrings, not to mention rings. Which latter items, by the way, are always worn on the far side of the wrists.

External healing, part 2: Externalization of diseases:
Yet for Blagrave, there is still more. With techniques I can only describe as astonishing, Blagrave is able to externalize ailments from the body entirely. Once removed from the body, ailments can be treated remotely, with great effect. Among these cures, the patient's own excrement is used to fertilize soil into which are planted the seeds of herbs which will cure. Another method is to take puss from an abscess, insert it into a hole drilled in a tree, close the hole, and let the tree do the healing. He gives a formula for Sympathetical Powder (pg. 133) which, when brought into contact with blood or puss removed from the patient, heals the patient, even though it was not at any time in contact with the patient himself.

Blagrave gives the name Sympathetic Cures to these methods, but I might liken them to cures by siphoning, as, in every case, the external method of healing in fact siphons the diseased material from the body, until none is left. This is not only powerful, but revolutionary, and deserves an impartial and fair investigation.

Casting out devils:
In organizing the Index I confess I largely ignored Blagrave's handling of devils and those possessed by them. This was in part as I doubt his methods were much better than those employed in modern times (shout at it until you have shouted it away), and because I myself know of superior methods. These methods require both innate skill, as well as intensive training and, as such, are not likely to become commonplace.

In the 1990's, I was trained in Pranic Healing, which was popularized by the Filipino, Choa Kok Sui. Among the various techniques in this method, the hands - which, remember, are sensitive to energies in the environment - are used to "imaginatively" "scoop" diseased matter from the body, which is then flung into a bucket of heavily salted water, known as a bioplasmic disposal unit. Various workers have various ideas what this diseased matter looks like. To me, it appears like clay slip, which is a very thin soup of clay. To my wife, it appears like dry gravel. Siphoning the material would have been easier than clawing it out, I think.

Editor's Preface: Witches and devils

An extension of the Pranic technique involves imagining the hands to be of various colors, white-whitish green being one of them. These colors/energies, abundantly present on the planet, enter the healer's body through his various chakras (each of which is qualified by one or another color), so that the energies the healer uses are determined by the state of his chakras and their ability to draw energy from the surrounding environment. There is an interesting annex to this theory, when the healer transmits energy through his crown chakra, which is located at the very top of his head. Viewed psychically, this energy appears very much like flashbulbs set off in your face, in other words, so bright it looks black. While the healer is generating and using this energy, there is a strong burning sensation at the very top of his head, which reminds one of the descent of the Holy Ghost upon the Apostles, the Holy Ghost being represented by flame. Using his hands, the healer pounds this energy into the patient's solar plexus, where it breaks addictions, such as that to tobacco or drugs. Which I have twice seen demonstrated, and which I myself once did. A powerful healer can do the work in thirty minutes. I took an hour, and was guided by a clairvoyant.

It is said this technique, known as Pranic Psychotherapy, will cast out spirits. As it works directly on hardened matter in and around the solar plexus chakra, I know of no reason why this would not be true. I mention it here as, while it is tiring, it is far less taxing than Blagrave's method. For skeptics who disbelieve in spiritual possession, I remind them that multiple personality disorder is, in fact, the modern term, and that descriptions of those so afflicted will exactly match those given by Blagrave.

<u>Witchcraft</u>:

Which brings me to witches and witchcraft. I was going to go along with popular consensus, that the sort of witches that Blagrave railed against no longer exist, or if they do, that they are rare and unlikely to trouble anyone overmuch.

But then, while browsing about the web a month ago, I came across a first-hand account by someone who, while not calling herself a witch, was using what amounted to sorcery and witchcraft to ensnare a lover. She was explicit about her technique, presumably unaware of how a knowing operator could easily turn her spell against her, and how dangerous that would be to her.

So I will tell you this. The sort of people who Blagrave describes still exist. They publish books detailing their techniques. You will not find such books on the same shelf where you found this one. You will not find them in the same store. You will not find them in any store in your neighborhood. (The books you will find, claiming to be "true witchcraft" are nothing of the sort.)

To find the real books on witchcraft, you must go to neighborhoods where, in fact, you never go. You must seek out stores that do not in any way resemble a bookstore. Like as not you will only ever visit such neighborhoods while on holidays or vacation, and your time there will be brief, because it will be most foreign to you. Should you, by some fantastic chance, happen to be in such a neighborhood and wander into such a store, you will be expecting something quite different from the books of magic and witchcraft on the shelves. Like as not you would not recognize such books even if you opened them. Such is how witchcraft keeps itself apart. Now as well as in Blagrave's day. Once you know what to look for, you will find such stores easily and without the slightest problem.

There are people today who claim that witches were wise old women who, at worst, burned candles and held simple rituals. It is claimed these unfortunates were tragically misunderstood. I regret to say that nothing in Blagrave's book - or in Lilly's - supports this claim.

Blagrave makes a distinction between witchcraft and sorcery. Witchcraft he defines as making a small model, or doll, of a specific person, and then sticking a pin in it, in order to cause torment to the victim. We now term this "voodoo", but that trivializes various west African/Caribbean religions. Sorcery Blagrave defines as injecting some evil matter into the person's body, by unspecified (and unknown to me) magical means. This can result in any disease whatever, which is why it was so critically important to get the right ascendant in the decumbiture chart, so that the true state of the twelfth house could be known.

Specifically, in the case on pgs. 127-9, where a minister put a prepared substance in a drink, thereby casting a spell upon his victim, we know this substance was not a poison or a disease, as the terms are understood, because poisons and diseases work on specific areas of the body over a given period of time, leading to a crisis from which the person either recovers, or dies. Whatever was afflicting the woman, Blagrave's description makes it clear her enormous weight gain was no ordinary ailment.

Ailments caused by witches or sorcerers could only be cured by first neutralizing the witch responsible. Blagrave's method, which is identical to Lilly's, involves taking the urine or blood of the victim, and then burning it up in a fire. The reason this works, as Blagrave explains, is that the witch had infected the victim with some essence of herself. This essence was present in the victims's blood and was discharged in the urine, so when the urine was destroyed, the essence of the witch trapped in it was destroyed along with the urine. By sympathy, or by siphon, burning the polluted urine caused the essence of the witch to be drained from her, resulting in her demise.

Was this nice? No, it was not. Could it lead to the witch's death? By Blagrave's and Lilly's express statements, yes, it could. If so, was that death fair, or just? This point is debateable. There is the matter of self-defense. It may be that the witch did not mean to cause death, merely torment, therefore a method of healing that causes her death would be unjustifiable. On the other hand, because the witch had worked in secret, and because the ailment had no other remedy, it would be up to the witch to ensure that a healer not ensnare her in this fashion, at the risk of her life.

We know that the destruction of a sample of one's own blood or urine does not cause harm or death to anyone, as various modern medical tests can result in such destruction. But if, on the other hand, the burning of blood or urine does lead to another person being harmed, or even loosing his life, then we may presume the existence of malevolent witches to be confirmed. Despite popular beliefs to the contrary.

Prayer:

Blagrave, and many others, recommended prayer to ward off the evils of witchcraft. Blagrave even went so far as to stake his fee on the report of his newly-cured patient, if they had prayed or not on the day they were afflicted. To modern ears this sounds like proselytizing, but it was nothing of the sort.

Just as there were malevolent energies that could cause harm, there are also reservoirs of beneficial energies that can protect from harm, if the individual wishes to make them available to him. This has long been one of the major claims of all religions, that there is a "God in Heaven" whose name, alone, once invoked, was sufficient to ward off evil.

In reality, this power was dependent upon the beliefs of the person making the plea, the construction of the prayer itself, and the intensity and focus with which it was uttered.

For example, the classic, "Now I lay me down to sleep, I pray to God my soul to keep" is clear, simple, direct, and employs both meter and rhyme. All of which enables the supplicant to put a great deal of hope and faith behind the utterance. (For best effect, prayers must be spoken aloud.)

By contrast, "Dear God, why me?", while frequently heard and always powerfully uttered, is structurally worthless and therefore ineffective.

Because a prayer that expresses one's own, unique, heartfelt needs and desires is better than a rote recitation of Our Fathers and Hail Marys, and because "God", as a word or a person is, in fact, unnecessary, one may well invent his own deity, and he may base it upon a favorite parent, grandparent, aunt, uncle or even friend. The better he knows the person, the more whole-heartedly he trusts the person (alive or dead, it makes no difference), the better the results. Many years ago I myself invented a fictitious "Louie" to watch over me. In many ways I think of him as a big, jolly Jupiter. Which is another hint: Base your "god" on something larger than yourself. So far as astrology is concerned, Jupiter and Venus, being benefics, will work nicely. So will the Sun, if you're careful not to let him burn or overwhelm you.

Such prayers, like umbrellas in the rain, work up to a certain degree. They are not, nor will they ever be, resistant to the worst storms that life may bring, but they will ward off much nonsense, certainly including the casual witch, and, by so doing, put you in a stronger position when dealing with the heavier seas of life.

Bloody brandy:

One of Blagrave's "pretty secrets" concerns mixing a small

amount of freshly drawn blood with spirits of wine, which we know as brandy. Closely stoppered and kept in a warm dark place, this mixture is said to reveal the overall health of the individual from whom the blood was taken.

This is such a simple thing that I will take it as proven, though I myself have not made the experiment. (I am interested in hearing from those who have.) Note that Blagrave is not using alcohol as a mere preservative. He is explicitly saying there is more than that. Alcohol enables blood removed from the body to remain in contact with it, and reflect changes in the body's overall health.

If this is true, it has a number of applications. Institutions with large numbers of people might use such samples as an easy check on the overall health of their residents. Schools and prisons come to mind. If precautionary samples were drawn, parents of runaways could know the relative health - or continued existence - of their missing children. Which would also be helpful for children at risk of being abducted, such as with custody battles. Those engaged in hazardous occupations, such as mining, manufacturing, working with infectious diseases, or, for that matter, prostitutes and drug addicts, could track the status of their own health, in real time. Athletes, or their managers, could use a sample to determine blood doping. Patients who must undergo radiation or chemotherapy could use a sample to monitor their overall health. Blagrave does not say how rapidly the extracted blood reacts to changes in body's health, but this could be easily established.

The science behind this neat trick is interesting. We start with the theory that we all live in an etheric / astral soup. This "fluid" connects us to each other. Thoughts and emotions flow through it, from one person to another, based on unwitting ability to send and receive.

The existence of this etheric substance has been doubted by traditional scientists, in part because, to date, there have been no conclusive tests that would reveal it. Bloody brandy might be what does.

And it would not be unprecedented. It has long been accepted that remnants of the motion of magnets and metals can be detected, at amazing distances, through the agency of a long loop of copper wire. We know this as electricity, but without the proper use of certain metals, and, critically, without a closed loop, the stream of current would not exist and electricity would be unknown. The needle of a compass is another analogy.

Since we know that blood, by itself, quickly perishes when taken from the body, the addition of alcohol seems to enable it to retain a mysterious contact with the host body and so not only remain alive, but also, if Blagrave is to be believed, react to subsequent changes in the host body. It is alcohol, presumably, which enables an essential contact to be made through the astral soup. This makes alcohol a sort of "copper wire". What can we do with this?

For starters, we can study the relative psychic ability between those who are perfectly sober, and the same people after they have ingested progressively greater amounts of booze. If Blagrave's observation is true, then psychic ability should increase when alcohol is present in the bloodstream, and not because the person is drunk, but, instead, because alcohol enhances contact, from one person to the next, through the astral ethers. Alcohol has long been the psychic's best friend, and that has long been a dirty little secret. Additionally, casual observation says that those who are slightly tipsy are more fun, less nervous, friendlier, "more connected", as it were. Which accounts for our nearly universal addiction to the drink.

Blagrave not only gives us a means of establishing the existence of the astral / etheric world, but a means of exploiting it. Blagrave also, inadvertently, explains some of the inner workings of witchcraft: The host who cast a spell over an unwitting guest by putting a mysterious powder in her drink. That drink, by definition, was alcoholic.

Severed hands:
Severed hands, the moss of a dead man's skull, a man's grease and more, are among the ingredients Blagrave uses. While macabre, it is less so than the elitist modern practice of harvesting organs from bodies only minutes dead.

<u>Inscriptions</u>:
Near the end of the book, Blagrave suggests wearing inscription as a means of healing. Success of such a method depends entirely upon the words chosen, and how the inscription is presented.

The analogy here is with educational degrees. Because of the way degrees are conferred upon graduates, various rights and powers are given as well as the scraps of paper. For this method to work, the words used must refer to some agreed-upon authority which cannot be questioned. It must be given by someone who has the authority to bestow the inscription. A doctor's prescription pad comes close to meeting these requirements.

Legality, fees:
Blagrave was often accused of using "illegal means" in his cures. Modern peoples seem to be less fussy. Close examination of Blagrave's methods, as I have done here, show them to be similar in many respects to those used by witches and sorcerers. But there are several notable differences:

The first is intent. Blagrave intends, hopes, and desires to make his patients well. A witch does not.

The second is the witch, but not Blagrave, uses her own organic materials upon her victims, in some mysterious way. Blagrave never does.

Third, the witch inflicts her "services" for "free", or appears to do so. In reality, what is "free" often comes with binding conditions, which, to this day, are frequently exploited by those offering their time, money, or services. We need only think of corporations who donate generously to politicians to understand the dangers of "free".

Blagrave, for his part, insists upon his fee, and while this sounds mercenary, it is nothing of the sort. Blagrave knows that healing that is not paid for will not work, and, also, that the expense of healing that fails is to be borne by the doctor alone. This is another way he distinguishes himself from other doctors, who insist on being paid whether they are successful or not. Blagrave's willingness to risk his income made him a better doctor. It gave him the incentive to study what worked, what did not, and to learn.

The source text:
The immediate source of this book was the 2001 facsimile printing by Ascella, a publisher which I believe no longer exists. It was of the first edition, of 1671. I believe Ascella's source to have been a

microfiche copy of unknown date and origin. This same microfiche is available on-line, as I had reason to compare it to my printed copy. The images of the two copies, Ascella and Google Books, matched precisely.

Pagination. Ascella used its own Arabic numbers for the title page, copyright page, table of contents, Dedicatory, and, To All My Loving Countrymen, ending at page 16. The Introductory Preface was not paginated by Ascella nor by the original printer in London. I have given all of this, along with this Preface, Roman numerals.

Proper Arabic pagination, in the original, the Ascella, and this edition, starts with A Catalogue of Herbs and Plants as page 1.

In the first edition there are these irregularities:

Pages 38 and 39 are missing, and the pagination of both Ascella, and the microfiche, are so arranged (even pages on the left, odd pages on the right) as to make one think the microfiche missed a facing page group, which is unlikely. More likely a leaf was missing from the copy used by the microfiche. I was able to find the missing text on-line, but it had been reset.

In this edition, the restored text can be found on pages 49-51, and is enclosed by [ ] at the beginning and ending.

In the Ascella, and the microfiche, what follows page 40 is page 73. In medieval books it was customary to put the first word of the next page on the last line of the proceeding page. This was for purposes of collation, as early books were printed as individual leaves which were collated manually. The last word on page 40, and the first on page 73, is Some. Which, as they match, indicates that Blagrave intended page 73 to follow immediately after page 40. In this edition, these are pages 52 and 53. I am grateful to Philip Graves, of Stockholm, who obtained a copy of the second edition of 1689. He reports all pagination problems to have been resolved, and that the end of the original page 40 is immediately followed by the text of the original page 73.

This would indicate problems with the original edition, leading to the deletion of 32 pages. At the time, type was set in rows and then locked down into frames. This made editorial corrections difficult, as individual type had to be physically removed before corrections could be made. Given how individual page frames were constructed, once pages were deleted, it may have been prohibitively

Editor's Preface: Notes on the source text

expensive to reopen subsequent frames to change the page numbers.

What could have been on the missing pages? Often in the book, Blagrave refers to the numerical values of specific herbs, urging us to get our numbers right. For example, marigolds are ruled by the Sun. The Sun has five numbers given to it (1, 3, 4, 10, 12, from page 25), but which of these, specifically, is given to marigolds? Could it be the missing pages were an herbal, giving the virtues of each plant, along with its specific number(s)?

In this regard, I note entry 132 in Gardner's Bibliotheca Astrologica, also known as A Catalogue Rasione of Works on the Occult Sciences, volume 2, Astrological Books (1911, reprinted, 1977, Symbols and Signs, Pasadena, California). The entry reads:

> **Blagrave** (Joseph) Blagrave's Supplement or Enlargement to Mr. Nich. Culpeper's English Physitian, containing a description of the Form, Names, Place, Time and Vertues of all Medicinal Plants as grown in England, &c. 8vo. London, 1674.

To which Gardner adds, "Collation (iv) 237 (xv) pp. Tract at end 46 pp." I should like very much to see this book in print. It may be that, faced with expenses he did not foresee, Blagrave deleted 32 pages of his herbal, perhaps because he had previously published a better version.

Continuing the pagination, in Ascella the page after 120 is numbered 137, but it has been crossed out and 121 written beside it. The text flows smoothly from one page to the next, as it does with the following gaps:

After page 137/121 comes pgs 122 and 123, and then (in this order) 140, 141, 126, 127, 144, 145, 130, 131 (manually renumbered 147), 148, 149, 134, 135, 152, 153, which is followed by pages in the normal order, ending at page 167.

Between 167 and 168 there is a gap. The end of page 167 ends with,

... I question not but that Authors have largely and learnedly written hereupon, unto whom I shall re-

Page 168 begins with,

I do seldom trust, or rely upon my judgement herein, . . .

Again my thanks go to Mr. Graves, who supplied the missing words from his edition of 1689: "refer myself ; for". This appears to be a simple typo in the first edition. It can be found, in [ ], on page 159 of this edition.

Pagination, from pgs 168, to the end of the main text on page 187 in the Ascella edition, is without problem. There follows two unpaginated pages, with the title, To all such who are Students, and well-Willers unto this most excellent Science of Astrology. The Ascella edition concludes with a poem by H. Pratt, in Latin. My Latin is nil, but this seems to merely praise the book. I have omitted it, as I could not have transcribed it correctly.

Spelling. Spelling irregularities have been noted. I believe there is a simple explanation. Typesetting was done by two individuals. One read the author's text, aloud. The other set what he heard, using the spelling and punctuation (and, most likely paragraph breaks) he thought proper. Every hour or two, they traded places. The two men were from different locales and each brought his own proper spelling. Such was what an author had to put up with.

To the best of my ability, I have copied Blagrave's use of *italics* CAPS, and astrological glyphs (these last are infrequent). I have also copied his punctuation and paragraph breaks, as much as I would have liked to have modernized both.

I have replaced hath with has, doth with does, unto with to, etc. I have replaced verbs that end with -eth (encreaseth, diminisheth, etc.) with their modern equivalents. I have replaced words such as fixt with fixed, agree'd with agreed. I have left Sagitary and Aquary alone. I rendered the following, "I did mix it with oyle of young Puppies" as "I mixed it with oil of young Puppies" (page 113 in this edition), in other words, I simplified verbs. I did this to make Blagrave's text legible to modern readers. We don't speak, read or write the same way that Blagrave did, just as he did not speak, read, or write as Chaucer did, though there are about as many years from Chaucer to Blagrave as there is between Blagrave and ourselves. I hope the results are satisfactory.

Editor's Preface: Credits, legend

Credits:

My thanks to Jane Ridder-Patrick, for her help with archaic herbal names and lore, and to Philip Graves for answering countless sundry queries on spelling, pagination, and translation. Any errors in this text are mine.

Most special thanks to Mr. Anthony Manzi, of London and Australia, who sent me a copy of Scan Soft's Omni Page Pro and the instructions to use it to make a new edition of this amazing book.

David R. Roell
Bel Air, Maryland
February 20, 2010

	Planets		Signs
☉	Sun	♈	Aries
☽	Moon	♉	Taurus
☿	Mercury	♊	Gemini
♀	Venus	♋	Cancer
♂	Mars	♌	Leo
♃	Jupiter	♍	Virgo
♄	Saturn	♎	Libra
⊕	Fortuna / Part of Fortune	♏	Scorpio
☊	North node	♐	Sagittarius
☋	South node	♑	Capricorn
℞	Retrograde	♒	Aquarius
		♓	Pisces

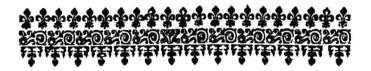

The Contents of this Book.

Editor's Preface	iii
To the truly learned and most Honoured Elias Ashmole	xxvii
To all my loving countrymen	xxix
A brief introductory Preface to the Reader	xxxiii

A Catalogue of the Herbs and Plants appropriate to the several Planets .... 1 - 6

General rules whereby to know under what planet every herb or plant is Governed .... 7 - 12

Rules concerning the gathering of herbs and plants at the right planetary hours .... 13 - 23

Concerning numbers attributed to the planets with the reason thereof .... 24 - 26

The way to find the Disease by the Sun or Moon afflicted .... 27 - 29

To know the time of Death or Recovery by the Critical Figure .... 30 - 31

Judgment upon a Decumbiture Figure, and also upon acute and perperacute sicknesses .... 32 - 34

Judgment upon another Decumbiture of a sick person .... 35 - 37

The Characters of the seven Planets : Twelve Signs ; and the five usual Aspects ; and the houses of the Planets .... 38 - 39

The sick-mans glass, with the use of an Ephemeris .... 39 - 41

How to Erect a Scheme or Figure for any time given .... 41 - 42

A Decumbiture Figure set for the time of my Friend's falling sick : with judgment thereupon .... 43 - 50

The Contents of this Book

Observations concerning the Ascendant .... 50 - 52

Brief Rules concerning long or short sicknesses and
    whether the Patient is like to live or die .... 53 - 56

The bodily shape and infirmities attributed to the twelve Signs .. 56 - 59

The bodily shape with the parts and members of the body
    together with the diseases which the planets generally rules .... 59 - 61

Concerning the Moon of Mars or Sol afflicted in any
    of the Twelve Signs .... 62 - 66

Concerning the Moon of Saturn or Jupiter afflicted
    in any of the Twelve Signs .... 66 - 70

How to make Diet-drinks, or to extract the spirits of
    plants or Herbs. How to make Syrups, Lambatives,
    Glisters, Fumes, Fumigations, Cataplasms,
    Ointments, and Baths .... 71 - 77

Of Purgations and the manner of Purging, Vomiting,
    Bathing, Sweating, Blooding, with some other
    additions necessary to be known .... 77 - 81

A Catalogue of Choice herbs or plants, collected for the curing
    of all kinds of griefs or infirmities whatsoever,
    Alphabetically expressed, beginning at .... 82 - 109

One cure done at Oxford, Anno Dom. 1658 .... 110 - 111

Another cure done at Oxford, Anno Dom. 1659 .... 112 - 115

One cure done at Tylehurst near Reading, Anno 1667 .... 115 - 116

The way to cure the Evil, commonly called the King's Evil;
    with an Example. Another kind of Evil and the
    Cure thereof .... 117 - 127

Another kind of Evil which comes from Strong Sorcery
    or Witchcraft with the way of cure .... 127 - 129

A Boy suddenly struck dumb and so continued three
    years how cured .... 129 - 132

How to make the Sympathetical powder with its application .. 133 - 135

The Contents of this Book

The Unguent its making and use .... 136 - 137

Concerning Witchcraft and Sorcery, with the way of cure .... 137 - 140

Some experimental Rules whereby to afflict the Witch .... 141 - 143

The way to cure both Witchcraft and Sorcery .... 143 - 144

Some notable Philosophical Secrets whereby to
    cure sundry distempers .... 145 - 148

Two pretty secrets in Philosophy .... 149 - 150

Some practical and experimental Rules whereby to
    give judgment Astrologically upon Thefts, Strays,
    Fugitives, Decumbitures of Sick Persons, Urines,
    or any other Horary Question .... 150 - 159

Concerning the casting forth of Devils out of such who are
    Possessed, and how performed by the Author .... 159 - 169

Concerning Agues and Quotidian Infirmities with the way
    of cure thereof .... 169 - 178

Concerning all kinds of Madness, its cause and cure .... 179 - 183

Postscript to the Reader : A short Epistle to those who
    are Students and well willers to the Art of Astrology ..... 184 - 185

<u>Appendices</u>:
    List of herbs .... 189 - 193
    The Pre-Copernican World 194
    Table of Essential Dignities 195
    Azimene degrees 195
    Temperament, *excerpted from* Astrological Judgement
        of Diseases from the Decumbiture of the Sick,
        by Nicholas Culpeper .... 196 - 203
    Glossary .... 203 - 215
    Extract from Smith's Family Physician, *on agues* .... 216 - 218
    Bibliography .... 219 - 220

Index 221

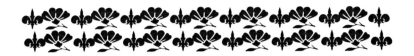

To the truly Learned, and my most Honoured
Friend *Elias Ashmole* of the *Middle
Temple* Esq; *Windsor* Herald at
Arms, and Comptroller of
the Excise for his
MAJESTY.

SIR,

Although somewhat abashed (when I confider those admirable gifts both of Learning and Knowledge which are seated in your worthy Person as by your admirable works in Print are manifest) to Dedicate these my Labours, yet being emboldened not only by our former acquaintance, as having ever found those noble parts in you, both of Wisdom and Affability : but also considering the great love and affection you did always bear to Philosophy : and so by consequence, a true lover of such, who are well-willers thereunto, according to that Maxim in Philosophy, Every thing delights in its own Element, and does sooner adhere to it, than to its contrary : and should this Book come into some men's hands who are not delighted in these kinds of Studies, although wise and well learned in other things, yet they will assuredly slight, and not regard what I have written, nor yet willingly show any love or countenance to the Writer, for according to that notable expression of yours to the Reader, in your excellent Book, entitled, The way to Bliss : That 'tis as possible to shape a Coat for the Moon, as in writing to please every Genius : so various are the generality of our inclinations, &c. What I have written in this Book is no Translation, but merely the subject of my many years Practice and Experience in the Astrological way of Physick : and Published, not only for my own vindication in point of Art and Practice, but also to instance others to do the like Cures as I have done ; for I may truly say, by me Wonders have been wrought, as in this Book will appear : yet many people I find are unsatisfied concerning my way of practice in Physick, the reason I conceive is, because many illiterate persons, and others who are ignorant of the Art of Astrology do foolishly speak against it, verifying that notable saying of the Poet Ars non habet inimicum nisi ignorantem. Concerning the lawfulness of the Art, I have sufficiently given satisfaction to the wise, in the Epistles of those Almanacs of mine, Dated Anno, 1658 and 1659. Besides, there are many excellent Men who have written both learnedly and largely thereupon ; should I mention your most worthy self, who is known to be a great Master herein, and not only in Astrology but also in Philosophy, the most excellent part having I dare say, few or no equals living. Sir, for the love I bear to your most Worthy Person, and to those most excellent gifts which God has endowed you with, I heartily wish I had higher and more excellent things to present you, that so you might take delight in reading, and increase in Knowledge thereby : however, I question not, but that when you have read it over, you will find somewhat herein worthy your perusal which may (if add nothing to your wisdom and Knowledge) put you in mind of greater Mysteries : even as in Motions, the lesser wheels being moved, causes the greater wheels to be set on work. Craving pardon for the boldness of him who heartily wishes your increase, both in Celestial, and Terrestrial Wisdom, Health, and Happiness in this Life, and Eternal Joy in the Life to come ; and who shall ever remain,

       Sir, Your assured Friend and
        Servant to Command

          Jos. Blagrave.

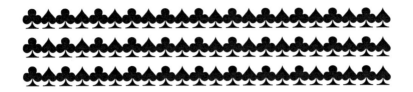

To all my loving Country-men in general, but especially to those of Reading, being the place of my Nativity.

IT *was the saying of our Blessed Saviour* That a Prophet could not be without honour save in his own Country. *Although I count myself no Prophet, yet by the Rules of* Astrology *I have predicted such things which (to our sorrow) have come to pass as may appear in my* Almanack *for the year* 1665 *and others formerly written : I presume, I have both Friends, and Enemies amongst you ; its well known to many, that I have done very great cures both in the Town, and places adjacent, although I have not mentioned their names in this Book, yet I find that many being unsatisfied concerning the legality of my way of Cure, have refused to come or send to me for help to cure their infirmities : and many of those who did come, came for the most part privately, fearing either loss of reputation or reproaches from their Neighbours, and other unsatisfied people ; and also fearing that what I did, was either Diabolical, or by unlawful means. I question not but when you have read over this Book, although some things may seem mystical at the first, especially to such who never before read any books of this nature, yet by oft perusal and well heeding what I have written, I am confident it may, and will give satisfaction to any of reasonable capacity and for the benefit of those who desire Knowledge in the Astrological and Chymical way of Physick (which is the most assured way extant) I have both briefly and plainly instructed the learner herein, so that those who can but read and will take pains may assuredly attain to it, and be enabled thereby to do the like Cures* as I have done : and as concerning the resolution of questions by Figures, a thing much questioned by some, I have in this book given sufficient reasons thereof according to Art, thereby enabling others (if they please to take the pains) to do the like. What I have formerly done herein, was more to satisfy the earnest importunity of others, than for any gain or profit which came to me, for I always (although some reward was given me for my pains therein) accounted myself a loser thereby, in regard of my Practice in Physick ; and let the Artist be never so careful to give content, yet what will the most men say, (especially such who are ignorant of the Art) if we discover the thing sought after, surely he does it by the Devil, otherwise, how could he do it, but if we chance to fail, as sometimes we may by taking a wrong Ascendant, then they will assuredly say, they are cheated of their money : I speak seriously. I take no pleasure in such questions, for the reasons aforesaid, having denied many which came to me therefore. Kind Country men and Women, my thoughts are better of you than wholly to blame you, for I dare say it was either false reports, or ignorance of the way I profess, which caused many of you to be inimical to me ; wherefore, I have the rather published this Treatise that so for time to come, you may not only be settled in your opinion, but also be fully satisfied, that what I have already done, or shall for time to come do in the Astrological or Chymical way of Physick, which is the way of my Practice, is both honest, just and lawful ; and is no more than what every industrious Physician ought to know, and without knowledge therein, its impossible to be an expert Physician, as in this book will appear : Concerning the Legality of this Art of Astrology, if any are unsatisfied they may read my Epistles of those Almanacks Dated, 1658 and 1659 besides there are many Authentic Authors who have written both learnedly and largely thereupon, for I intend not at this time to trouble myself or reader much farther herein, only this much at present, I say, next to Divinity it is the most to be admired and most excellent study in the World, and worthy our Knowledge ; for there is so much seen of the wonderful Work of God in it, that it must needs convince the most unbelieving persons whatsoever, and cause them to know that a mighty and powerful hand has wrought

To all my loving Country-men.

those wonders which we visibly see, as the Heavens, Sun, Moon, Stars *and* Planets, *with their Motions and powerful Operations over all sublunary Creatures ; and has given to man so much Knowledge thereby (next to the Angels) that he is able to reveal and make known in a great measure his Heavenly Will thereby to his People, that so they may be forewarned of his wrath to come. If I find this Book has acceptance with you, I shall he encouraged to labour in my study and profession to do you and the Country further service, and shall ever remain, your assured loving Country man and Servant.*

Jos. Blagrave.

AN Introductory Preface TO THE READER

Having formerly spent some of my youthful years in the Study of *Astronomy* and *Astrology*; and since that, in *Philosophy* and the practice of *Physick*, and finding by good experience how each part depends upon the other, for without some knowledge in *Astronomy*, one can be no *Astrologer*; and without knowledge in *Astrology*, one can be no *Philosopher* and without Knowledge both in *Astrology* and *Philosophy*, one can be no good *Physician* and whosoever desires to make practice, either in the *Astrological* or *Chymical* way of Physick (as for the Drug way, there can be no certainty in curing thereby, as will plainly appear in this book) having laid his foundation as aforesaid (which if any Practitioner or Student in Physick be ignorant of, this Book will sufficiently instruct them therein) must build and rely upon these five substantial Pillars following, without which, there can be no admirable cures done or wonders wrought in this noble Art of Physick, *Viz*. Time, Virtue, Number, Sympathy and Antipathy. *First*, Time is of great Concern whereby to gather each Herb or Plant at the right Planetary hours, which this book will sufficiently inform you; and likewise to know the hour and time when to administer your Physick aright, for if the Physick be administered at a wrong hour, be it Purge or Vomit it will work contrary effects, as I have often times proved : *Example*, If you give a Purge when the *Moon* is in an Earthy Sign, Aspected by a Planet Retrograde, and that the Ascendant with its Lord Corresponds, then the Purge will turn to a Vomit : and on the contrary, if a Vomit be given when the *Moon* is in a Watery Sign, Aspected by Planets swift in Motion out of Watery Signs, the Signs Ascending with its Lord Corresponding, then the Vomit will turn to a Purge : also an exact time must be obtained whereby to erect your Figure aright, whereby to give judgment upon the disease, its cause and termination, which this book will sufficiently instruct you in. For by Urine alone, no true judgement herein can be given, except in some few infirmities which proceed from the blood, or passages of Urine, for Urine is but the excrement of blood : there are many other considerations to be made use of by virtue of time, which I for brevity's sake am willing at present to pass over, and so shall proceed to the word Virtue, which is in brief, a right knowledge and understanding of the Nature, Properties, Elemental Qualities and Effects which each Herb or Plant has, whereby to cure all kinds of griefs or infirmities whatsoever, either by Sympathy or Antipathy, as this book will sufficiently inform you ; and all growing within our Nation. I shall not trouble myself or Reader in setting forth the dangers in using foreign Drugs, yet I deny not, but that some Drugs, whose virtue and operations are well known to us may in many respects be useful, by reason our Climate does not afford some ingredients which are necessary to be used in some Distempers, as Figs, Raisins, Currants, Sugar, Wine, and Spirits &c. which are often times made use of, whereby to make our Diet-drinks and spirits of Plants extracted the more savory, and helps to work a more forcible effect in many distempers, as you will find in this book : and I have accordingly in some infirmities made use thereof.

Thirdly, concerning *Number* : there are certain Numbers attributed to the Planets, which every Astrological or Chymical Physician ought to know ; more especially, such who use this way of cure by Herbs or Plants which is the most assured way extant as best agreeing with our *English* bodies, yet as I have already declared both in Decoctions, and in Chimical Extractions, Ingredients, together with Herbs may be used to make it the more forcible and savory ; but should we take all Herbs or Plants which are accounted good for every grief, not having regard to any select Number, there being so many sorts of Herbs approved good for the same, there would be no certainty either for the gathering of the Herbs at a right hour, or yet know when you have enough whereby to work your cure : the certainty of a select Number is not only according to my own experience, but also its the Opinion of *Cornelius Agrippa*, an excellent Philosopher, and many others : What Numbers are attributed to each Planet, and the reasons thereof, I have elsewhere in this book expressed.

Fourthly, Concerning *Sympathy*, that is, when any Planet who is strongest in the Heavens by essential dignities, shall afflict the Principal significator of the sick, especially, if more strong than that Planet which is of a contrary nature ; then those herbs or Plants which are under his Dominion, shall according to their Virtues and Numbers be collected to cure the infirmity, always provided, they are gathered at the right Planetary hours, which this Book will inform you ; *Example*, If *Mars* be the afflicting Planet and is more strong in essential dignities than *Venus*, then you must make choice of such Herbs which are under the dominion of *Mars* to cure such infirmities which he usually produces, which this Book will also acquaint you with. There is no infirmity or disease whatsoever, but in a second Cause proceeds from the evil influence of the afflicting Planets ; and what infirmity soever any Planet causes, he has Herbs by Sympathy to cure it : in this condition, heat must fetch out heat, even as if one should burn one's Finger, and then heat it against the fire, which cures by Sympathy: Likewise, I have known a great cold taken, to be cured by a Pippin taken in cold water, *Venus* being strong in essential dignities; and if we should give cooling remedies when *Mars* is strong, it will destroy the Patient, as I have often proved ; for it stands by reason, that if a weak man contend with a strong man well armed, he must needs be worsted : but if *Mars* be the afflicting Planet, although strong, and *Venus* also be near equal in strength, then we must choose a select lesser Number of her herbs to join with *Mars*, and so the dose must be proportioned according to their strength and weakness, and so the remedies will be between both, rather adhering to the strongest Planet.

Fifthly, Concerning *Antipathy*, admit the *Moon* or principal Significator of the sick be afflicted by *Saturn*, a Planet Cold and Dry, and he weak in the Heavens, and the Planet which is of a contrary nature is strong, as instance *Jupiter* who is Hot and Moist, then a select Number of Herbs under the dominion of *Jupiter*, being of virtue to cure the distemper must be used, provided they are gathered at the hour when *Jupiter* reigns, which this book will inform you. But if *Saturn* and *Jupiter* be near equal in strength, then use a medium between both, and let one part of your Herbs be by Sympathy under *Saturn*, and the other part under *Jupiter*, always adhering to the stronger Planet, both by Number and Dose, and ever remembering in all Cures whatsoever to use a select number of Herbs which are under the *Sun*, in regard he is Fountain of Life, and sole Monarch of the Heavens ; and all those Herbs which are under his Dominion are always approved good to comfort the Heart, Brain, Nerves, Arteries, and Vital Spirits, and are likewise good to resist Poison : Likewise in all Cures whatsoever, you must have regard to the age of the Patient, together with their Complexion, and the season of the year, that so you may help to support Nature's defects, for a Choleric or Sanguine Man or Woman by nature requires things more cooling than Phlegmatic, or Melancholy Man or Woman, and a Phlegmatic or Melancholy man or woman requires things more heating than a Choleric or Sanguine man or woman ; consider the like between Youth and Age, and the season of the year. *Note*, that each herb or plant mentioned in this Treatise, is set down by way of Catalogue under the *Planet* which owns the Plant or Herb, it being done according to their Elemental Qualities and Virtues : Having given sufficient reasons thereof, I confess I much differ from Authors, for what I have written in this book is no Translation, being merely according to my Practice and Experience for many years, by virtue of which Herbs and plants (through God's blessing) I have done many great and wonderful cures, I dare say, greater has not been done since the Apostles' times, for I have caused the blind to see ; the deaf to hear ; both lame and bedridden people to go ; the dumb to speak ; such who have been in extremity of pain, I have eased them ; likewise I have cured all kinds of Evils, and all kinds of Agues ; together with all sorts of Madness, having in this Book given sufficient reasons for the same : I have likewise inserted in this Book ; the Names, and places of dwelling of sundry persons who have been by me cured of such infirmities and griefs aforesaid, and how performed ; that so others may be informed how to do the like : I have also instructed the Learner, how by the *Moon* in acute, or *Sun* in Chronic griefs, or infirmities to find the disease with its cause, and termination. I have also shown the way how to Erect a Figure, and thereby to give judgment, either upon the Decumbiture, sight of the Urine or any strong fit of the Patient. And for the benefit of such who desire further inspection into this Art of *Astrology*, having by the Rules in this Book, or by their own study attained to the perfect way of Erecting a Figure : I have shown the way how to give judgment upon any horary question, as Thefts, Strays, Fugitives, and Urines, &c. it being according to my way of Practice and Experience for many years.

I have also shown the way and manner how I have cast forth Devils, out of such who were possessed, that so others may be informed to do the like.

Courteous Reader, what I have written in this Book, is not only for my own vindication against all scandals and false aspersions which are usually cast upon me, by such who are ignorant of my way of Practice, but chiefly to instruct others, and to enable them to do the like Cures I have done, that so many hundreds may be kept from perishing. There are many who admire at the Cures by me done, but being unsatisfied of the Legality of my way of Cure, thereupon refuse to come, or send to me for help, to cure their infirmities.

And as for the vindication of the Art of *Astrology*, I shall not at present trouble myself or Reader therewith, but shall refer those who are unsatisfied; to those Epistles in my Almanacs, Dated *Anno* 1658 and 1659 and to many other authentic Authors in Print.

Some Observations Concerning Sympathy of Cure.

WHereas in the Catalogue of Plants, the Planet *Saturn* has but very few Herbs or Plants allotted to him : yet not withstanding in my Epistle before going, I told you, that what griefs or infirmities whatsoever any Planet caused, there are herbs by Sympathy, as well as Antipathy to cure it; wherefore know that, although an Herb or Plant may by Elemental qualities be under the Dominion of *Mars*, as being hot and dry, and so gathered at his hour, yet in regard of his virtues, and being approved good to cure such infirmities which are under the Dominion of *Saturn*, it may justly and rationally be called a Sympathetic Cure, by reason *Mars* is exalted in *Capricorn* the house of *Saturn*. *Example*, Agues, especially Quartans, are usually caused by *Saturn*. Now Wormwood, Carduus, and such like Plants being hot and dry, are properly attributed to *Mars*, both in point of gathering and numbers, yet in regard these Herbs and Plants are of known virtues to cure Agues which *Saturn* causes ; and *Mars* being exalted in *Capricorn* which is the house of *Saturn* : therefore it may properly be called a Sympathetic Cure : And so Herbs under the Dominion of *Sol*, cure infirmities by Sympathy caused by *Mars*, because the *Sun* is exalted in *Aries* the house of *Mars* : And so Herbs under *Venus* cure by Sympathy infirmities under *Jupiter*, by reason *Venus* is exalted in *Pisces* the house of *Jupiter* ; and so herbs of *Jupiter* cure by Sympathy such diseases which are under the dominion of the *Moon*, by reason *Jupiter* is exalted in *Cancer* which is her house : The benefit which we have from this observation is as follows ; If *Saturn*, *Mars* or any other Planet, be the afflicting Planet, and strong (which argues a Compliance) then those herbs which are under the dominion of that Planet which is exalted in his house, being good for to cure the infirmity may be used and (for the reason aforesaid) it shall be called a Sympathetic Cure, for when Planets are strong and afflicting we must comply with them, as I have elsewhere expressed. *Note*, that in all Sympathetic cures whatsoever, there must be one Elemental quality in the Planet of compliance, with the nature of the Planet afflicting ; as for Example, Herbs under *Mars* have the quality of dryness with *Saturn* ; and Herbs under the *Sun* have the quality of heat with *Mars*, and Herbs under *Venus* have the quality of moisture with *Jupiter*; And Herbs under *Jupiter* have the quality of moisture with the *Moon*.

The truth is, I find by good experience, especially in very cold infirmities, as Agues, Dead palsies, and such like, it's impossible to make a Sympathetic Cure when *Saturn* is strong, were it not so that those Observations before-going were in force, and approved : as for example, if the Patient be old, his grief cold, his Complexion cold, the season of the year cold, and his remedies to be applied cold, it must needs destroy nature, for where heat is wanting there can be no life : but if *Saturn* be the afflicting planet and weak then herbs which are under the dominion of the *Sun* and *Jupiter* being of known virtue to cure the Distemper or grief will do it ; they being by Nature hot and moist; whereas *Saturn* is by nature cold and dry, clean differing in Elemental qualities, and this is called an Antipathetical Cure ; but in all infirmities whatsoever which are caused by the evil influence of *Mars*, he being strong in the Heavens, the remedies used must be by such Herbs and plants which are under his own Dominion, together with herbs of the *Sun*, but if the Complexion of the patient, their age, and the season of the year naturally produces heat, then to use some small numbers and dose of such herbs which are under the Dominion of *Venus*, may be proper at some convenient times to give the patient towards the refreshing of nature, yet chiefly in point of Cure you must adhere to those herbs and plants which are under *Mars* and the *Sun* whereby to work your Cure, for if you should give cooling remedies in hot Distempers when *Mars* is strong, it will destroy the patient as I have sufficiently proved ; but as I have elsewhere expressed if *Mars* be the afflicting planet and weak, then those herbs and plants under the Dominion of *Venus* and the *Moon* ; together with a select number of Herbs under the Dominion of the *Sun* will do it.

In all Cures whatsoever, a select number of herbs under the dominion of the *Sun* must be used.

These Rules being well observed and carefully followed, may through God's blessing produce wonderful Effects ; as I have sufficiently proved in my many years practice and experience, as you will find in this Book.

BLAGRAV's Astrological Practice of Physick.

A CATALOGUE

Of the HERBS and PLANTS in this Treatise mentioned being rightly appropriated to their several Planets, according to their elemental qualities and virtues, and agreeing with the Author's experience and practice for many years : There are many other herbs, which might have been inserted herein, but these here mentioned are the most material and useful, being all English Plants and well known, and without question, if rightly applied, may well serve to cure any infirmities, whatsoever that are curable, as I have sufficiently proved. But those that please may insert others, having knowledge of their elemental qualities and virtues, according to the Rules hereafter expressed.

Saturn	Saturn	Jupiter
Alder-black	Moss of Oak.	Agrimony.
Bird's-foot.	Night shade	Alexanders.
Bulleys.	Oak.	Aromatical-reed.
Clown's woundwort.	Poppy-black	Beans-blue.
Cattail.	Polypodium of the oak.	Betony of the wood.
Hawkweed.	Tway blade, or two leaved-grass.	Bittany of the water.
Hemlock.		Borage.
Henbane.		Cinquefoil.
Mandrake.		

Jupiter	Jupiter	Mars
Camels hay.	Orach with blue flowers.	Bend weed.
Columbine with blue flowers.	Poppy with blue flowers.	Birthwort.
Cresses.	Periwinkle.	Bishop's weed.
Comfrey with bluish or purple flowers	Purple wort.	Bitter-sweet.
Bugloss.	Parsnip.	Blites, with red flowers,
Bugloss wild	Parsnip wild.	Box-tree.
Dodder of thyme, or of any other Jupiter plant.	Spleenwort.	Bramble.
Dog stones.	Satirion.	Brooklime.
Elm-tree leaves and bark.	Saracens confound.	Broom.
Fell-wort.	Scurvy-grass.	Butchers broom.
Feverfew.	Smallage.	Broom rape.
Flower-de-luce.	Thyme.	Bryony.
Fools-stones.	Mother of Thyme.	Buckthorn.
Foxgloves, with purple flowers.	Wild flax.	Butter-bur.
Fumitory.	*Mars*	Butter wort.
Goats-beard, or Joseph's flower	Agnus castus.	Carduus benedictus.
Gromwell, flowers and leaves.	Alehoof, or ground ivy.	Catmint.
Gander-gosse.	Anemony.	Coloquintida.
Hart's tongue.	Anet.	Charlock.
Hyssop.	Archangel, with red flowers.	Cotton-thistle.
Knot grass.	Asarabacca.	Cockle.
Larkspur with blue flowers.	Arsmart.	Crowfoot.
Mallows.	Asphodel.	Crosswort.
	Beans red.	Danewort.
	Beets red.	Darnel.
	Bell flowers.	Dittander.
		Dittany or paperwort.
		Dogs tooth.
		Dragons blood.
		Dove's foot.

A Catalogue of Herbs and Plants

Mars

Dropwort.
Dyer's weed.
Elder-buds.
Fern.
Filipendula.
Fleabane.
Furzbush flowers.
Galangal.
Garlic.
Germander.
Gladdon stinking.
Glasswort.
Goutwort.
Ground pine.
Heath.
Hellebore.
Helmet flower.
Horehound.
Hawthorn.
Hemp.
Hops.
Holly.
Horsetail.
Jack by the hedge.
Ivy.
Knapweed.
Louse berries.
Leeks.
Monkshood.
Mouse ear.
Mustard.
Herb mercury.
Hedge-mustard.

Mars

Nettles
Nep.
Onions.
Osmond royal | both
Osmond water | flags
Park-leaves, or
   Tudson
Poppy red flowers.
Pilewort
Pepperwort.
Radish.
Ragwort.
Rocket.
Rhubarb.
Bastard-rhubarb.
Rupturewort.
Saw-wort.
Savin.
Saxifrage.
Sciatica cresses.
Scabious.
Scorpion-grass.
Spurge.
Self heal.
Sene.
Shepherd's needle.
Shepherd's purse.
Sneezewort.
Soapwort.
Spearwort.
Solomon's seal.
Swallowwort.
Tamarisk.

Mars

Thistles.
Tarragon.
Toothwort, or
   dentary.
Our Lady's thistle.
Wake-robin.
Cuckoopint.
Wormwood.
Woadwaxen.
Woad.
Wal-wort.
Wood sage.

Sun

Alecost or
   costmary.
Angelica.
Anise.
Ash-tree.
Almonds.
All-good.
Avens.
Basil-street.
Birds eye.
Burnet.
Bugle.
Calamint.
Camomile.
Centaury.
Chervil, or sweet
   Cicely.
Celandine.

Sun

Clary.
Catmint.
Cowslips.
Comfrey with yellow flowers.
Crown imperial good for palsies.
Daffodils, or Daffydowndilly.
Dill.
Dittany.
Eglantine.
Elecampane.
Eye-bright.
Fennel.
Figwort.
Golden rod.
Gilly-flowers sweet.
Herbs ears.
Holly rose.
Higtaler flowers yellow with woolly leaves.
Saint Katherine's flower.
Saint John's wort.
Saint James' wort.
Ladies bedstraw with yellow flowers.
Juniper.
Lavender.

Sun

Lavender cotton.
Lady's mantle.
Lovage.
Lilies yellowish flowers.
Marigolds.
Marjoram sweet.
Maudlin sweet.
Masterwort.
May weed.
Melilot.
Mints garden.
Mistletoe.
Mugwort.
Motherwort.
Mullein.
One blade, or herb true love.
Oxlips.
Parsley.
Saint Peter's wort.
Palma bristi.
Penny royal.
Pimpernel.
Peony.
Roes red.
Rosa solis.
Rosemary.
Roses damask.
Rue
Saffron.
Sanicle.
Sage.

Sun

Samphire.
Sandalwood.
Scordium.
Setwal.
Savoy, summer.
Southernwood.
Sunflower.
Sundew.
Spignel.
Tansy.
Tree of life.
Tormentil.
Valerian.
Vervain.
Walnut leaves.
Woodbine flowers, or honeysuckles.
Wood rose.
Vipers bugloss.

Venus.

Adders-tongue.
Apples.
Arrach stinking.
Archangel, white-flowers.
Arrow head.
Artichokes.
Alkanet.
Barley.
Beans-white.

A Catalogue of Herbs and Plants

Venus.

Bears-breach.
Beech-leaves.
Blites-flowers white.
Beets white.
Bucks, horn plantain.
Cleavers, or Goosegrass.
Coltsfoot.
Columbines with white-flowers.
Crab tree.
Cherry-tree and fruit
Cranesbill.
Cudweed.
Comfrey roots.
Daisies.
Dandelion.
Ducks meat.
Elder-flowers.
Fleawort.
Pellitory.
Flixweed.
Groundsel.
Gourds.
Harts-ease or herb of the Trinity.
Herb Truelove.
Herb twopence, or money wort.
Houndstongue.

Venus.

Larks Spur, with white flowers.
Lilies with white flowers.
Maidenhair.
Moss on Apple-trees or crabtrees.
Mulberries leaves.
Navel wort.
Orach flowers white.
Peach flowers.
Pellitory of the wall.
Plantain.
Periwinkle, wild.
Pond weed.
Poppy flowers white.
Pauls betony.
Primrose.
Ribwort.
Roses white.
Rushes.
Sandalwood flowers, white.
Snakeweed.
Sorrel wood.
Sowthistle.
Stichwort.
Spinach.
Strawberries.

Venus.

Sycamore tree.
Throatwort, or bell flower.
Three leaved grass.
Turnip root.
Vine leaves.
Violets, leaves & roots.
Water cresses.

Mercury.

Alkanet.
All-good.
Barberries.
Blood-wort.
Bell flower.
Blue bottle.
Dog grass.
Endive.
Fluellin.
Liverwort.
Loosestrife.
Loose-wort.
Lungwort.
Meadowsweet.
Medlar tree.
Madder.
Millet.
Privet.
Quinces.
Succory.

Mercury.	Moon
Rampion.	Cabbage.
Sorrel-garden.	Chickweed.
Starwort.	Coleworts.
Whortleberries.	Cucumber.
Willow-tree.	Houseleek or
Wood bine-leaves.	fengreen.
Wild Tansy.	Lettuce.
Yarrow.	Melons
	Orpine.
	Pompions.
	Purslane.
	Moon wort.

General Rules to know under what Planet every Herb or Plant is governed by only the use of an Herbal, with the true reason thereof, according to the Author's experience and practice for many years ; as follows.

The first thing to consider, is to take notice of the Elemental Qualities of each Planet ; *viz.* whether hot and dry, hot and moist, cold and dry, or cold and moist, and of what degrees; as first, second, third or fourth. Secondly, we must by an Herbal find the nature or Elemental quality of the plants ; if you find that both the Planet and plant accord in Elemental qualities then we may conclude, that such an herb or plant is under such a Planet : for any reasonable Philosopher well knows, that every Element naturally sympathizes with its own like, even as the actions of men naturally sympathize with their complexion and condition of that Planet which has predominance over them, as I have elsewhere expressed.

Example ♄

Saturn is a Planet cold and dry in the third and fourth degree : Now by the Herbs I find, that hemlock, henbane, nightshade, and such like, are cold and dry in the third and fourth degree ; and therefore may justly be attributed to the Planet *Saturn*.

♃

Jupiter is by nature hot and moist : Now by the Herbal I find, that borage, mallows, and the herb or plant called dog-stones, are by nature hot and moist ; and therefore may justly be attributed to *Jupiter*.

♂

Mars is by, nature hot and dry in the third and fourth degree : Now by the Herbal I find, that carduus, wormwood, tobacco, rhubarb, hellebore, box, and such like, are all under the dominion of *Mars*, as being hot and dry in the third and fourth degree.

☉

The *Sun* is by nature hot and dry in the first and second degree, and near to the third ; Now by the Herbs I find, that angelica, balm, marigolds, rue, sweet marjoram, and such like, are all hot and dry in the first and second degree, perhaps near to the third ; and therefore are all attributed to the *Sun*.

♀

Venus is by nature cold and moist in the first and second degree : Now by the Herbal I find, that violets, spinach, white beets, white beans, and such like, are all under the dominion of *Venus*, as being cold and moist in the first and second degree accordingly.

☿

Mercury is by nature cold and dry in the first and second degree: Now by the Herbal I find, that endive, succory, woodbine, lungwort, liverwort, and such like, are all cold and dry in the first and second degree, and are therefore under the dominion of *Mercury*.

☽

The *Moon* is by nature cold and moist in the third and fourth degree ; and by the Herbal I find, that cabbage, fengreen, chickweed, orpine, purslane, and such like, are all cold and moist in the third and fourth degree ; and therefore are under the dominion of the *Moon*.

Another way whereby to attribute each herb or plant aright to the Planet, that so they may agree both in elemental qualities and virtues, more especially of the first part in the degrees of heat or cold, it being the way of my practice, and that with good success.

First, having by an Herbal found the virtue of the plant which is approved for the curing of such infirmities or diseases which are under the dominion of such a planet, as causes them, although the herb or plant agree but in the first elemental quality of heat or cold, yet the herb or plant may justly and rationally be attributed to the Planet which owns the grief, and so thereby make a sympathetic cure : As instance, *Jupiter* who is by nature hot and moist, and has predominance over the liver, lungs, blood, veins, pleurisies, and the like : Now by the Herbal we find, that lungwort, wood-betony, agrimony, scurvy-grass, and such like, are all good to cure such infirmities, notwithstanding they are all hot and dry in the first and second degree, yet having the first elemental quality of heat, together with virtue to cure such defects which *Jupiter* causes, they may justly be attributed to *Jupiter* ; and so plantain, white beets, and dandelion, accounted by Authors cold and dry, may justly be attributed to *Venus*, as having the first elemental quality of being cold in the first or second degree, and has virtue to cure by sympathy such defects which *Venus* causes, or otherwise by antipathy to *Mars*, as does plantain, which cures cuts and wounds which *Mars* causes : Now white beets and dandelion cure by sympathy ; the first brings down women's courses, the other helps to cleanse the passages of urine, always provided in these particular applications, that the first elemental quality of heat or cold agrees, as aforesaid, without which there can be no true gathering or attributing the plant aright to the Planet, as I have shown more at large elsewhere. And further, should we not sometimes use this particular way herein expressed, both *Jupiter* and *Venus*, who are great friends to Nature, would have very few herbs or plants allotted to them, especially *Jupiter* who is the greater fortune ; for by the Herbal you shall find very few herbs or plants which accord in elemental qualities of heat and moisture with *Jupiter* ; and the truth is, I find that Authors most of them agree in the first elemental quality, or part of heat or cold, but in the latter part of dryness or moisture somewhat differing ; and without question they but guess thereat, or otherwise by tradition follow each other ; neither do they give true knowledge therein (especially in many herbs and plants) as instance dandelion, which has a known virtue to open and cleanse the passages of urine : Now if this plant were cold and dry, which most Authors hold, how could it have this virtue to open and cleanse ? for of necessity moisture must do it, for all plants which are drying, are usually stopping and binding ; and so *Saturn*, a Planet cold and dry, when afflicting the ☽ in earthy signs, always produces bindings in the body : Also the blossoms of plants are somewhat to be regarded, more especially when they agree in the first elemental quality of heat or cold ; as instance, wood-betony, hyssop, bugloss, borage, and such like, whole blossoms are blue, a colour which ♃ owns : And notwithstanding, they are all hot and dry (except borage) yet they are rightly appropriated to *Jupiter*, by reason of their virtues, as curing such defects which ♃ causes. But should we grant that herbs and plants, which are by Nature cold and dry, to be under *Jupiter* (as many learned Authors hold, as I could name) as instance endive, succory, and such like, there can be no reason given for it, by reason they are so much different in elemental qualities, for the plants are cold and dry, and the Planet *Jupiter* hot and moist, clean opposite to each other; wherefore it stands by reason, and is rational to be under *Mercury*, whose nature sympathizes, as being cold and dry, and so to cure by antipathy to *Jupiter*, the herbs being of known virtue to cure such distempers, which *Jupiter* causes; likewise I find that many Authors attribute, clary, mints, pennyroyal, and many others, to *Venus* a planet cold and moist, whereas the herbs are all hot and dry, of a clean contrary nature. Now these plants do properly belong to the *Sun*; and the rather in regard of their virtues, as being comfortable to the heart and vital spirits, and being of sweet smell, and pleasant taste: I could instance many more, which Authors wrongfully apply, as instance they attribute angelica, sage, box, and such like to be under the planet *Saturn* whereas the herbs are all hot and dry; especially box who is hot and dry in the fourth degree, both the first plants are without question under the dominion of the *Sun*, as being of a good smell and taste, and are of known virtues to comfort the heart, arteries, and vital spirits and to resist poison. The other being very hot, and of bitter taste rightly belongs to the planet *Mars* as agreeing in elemental qualities. I confess, I have read many Authors, and I find many of them accord, but clean out of the way of truth: The reason is, as I conceive, because their works are many, or most of them but translated, and so following by tradition each other, not well weighing the reasons have likewise erred, but as to the virtues of herbs and plants they do for the most part accord, giving reasons for the same. What I have written in this Book is not by imitation of others, but from my own daily practice and experience. And should I set down the many difficult cures, which I have done by virtue of herbs, I should hardly be believed, except by such who are well versed in the secrets of Astrology and Philosophy: for many country people think, they make a bold adventure, when they come to me for cure, presuming that what I do is more than natural. They not considering, or at least being ignorant of the extraordinary virtue of herbs and plants more especially being gathered at the right planetary hours together with the right numbers of herbs and plants belonging to each planet being collected and being truly in due times administered ; for time, virtue, and number, together with the right understanding of the way of cure by sympathy and antipathy are the principal pillars of our work in the Astrological or Chymical study of physick, as I have already declared in my before Epistle to the Reader.

Gathering of Plants and Herbs

Here follows some necessary Rules to be observed concerning the gathering of each herb or Plant aright according to the true planetary hours, without which no great cures can be done or wonders wrought in the Astrological and Chymical way of Physick. I have also set down the way how to reconcile any difference, which may sometimes arise by way of application of the plant to the planet: For I must confess by reason of the difference amongst Herbalists concerning the qualities and virtues of some particular plants there may happily be some rational contest therein.

The Way to gather such Herbs and Plants which are of known Elemental qualities and virtues out of contest is as follows

BEfore we proceed herein it will be necessary for the Reader to understand the planetary hours ; which are inserted at the beginning of the second Book together with the Almanack perpetual adjoining, for both the planet, which is Lord of the hour and the plant which is to be gathered must both agree in elemental qualities especially of the first part of heat or cold. *Example*, If I were minded to gather balm, rosemary, marigolds, angelica, and such like plants or herbs, which are under the dominion of the Sun ; upon *Sunday* the fourteenth of *March* 1669. Now from the *Sun's* rising until he is an hour in height which is until seven o'clock, is the hour of the *Sun*, likewise the *Sun* reigns again the eighth hour, which is between one and two o'clock after upon. At which times you may gather any herbs or plants under the dominion of the *Sun*. Now if any one were minded to gather any herbs of the *Sun* upon Tuesday the sixteenth day then between seven and eight o'clock in the morning is the hour of the *Sun*. And likewise between two and three o'clock afternoon, as appears in the Almanack answerable to the day of the Month, also by the same Rules you may gather any other Herbs or Plants at the right planetary hours accordingly, which are out of controversy.

Rules whereby to gather such Herbs and plants, which are in Controversy, that so you may have the true planetary influence notwithstanding as follows

When you are minded to gather any herb or Plant in controversy, as instance dandelion before mentioned, this Plant being by my rules under *Venus*, but by some Authors appropriated to *Jupiter* by reason it has a virtue to open the obstructions of the Liver (being under *Jupiter*). But it has also a virtue to open and cleanse the passages of urine, as I have already declared (which is under *Venus*) but chiefly it has the first elemental quality of being cold, agreeing with *Venus*, whereas *Jupiter* is hot. Now to reconcile this or any other difference of the like nature, do as follows : Let both Planets in question at the time of gathering be in *Conjunction*, *Sextile* or *Trine*, aspect to each other. Or otherwise let the *Moon* be separating and applying by any of those aspects from the one planet to the other, by this rule you may have the true planetary influence of both planets in question : Always provided that the Lord of the Hour accords with the first elemental quality of the planet be it hot or cold, wherefore in this condition *Venus* must be Lord of the Hour at the time of gathering the herb or plant accordingly. I shall instance one herb more ; Suppose, I was minded to gather Sweet-marjoram, which plant is by many Authors appropriated to the planet *Mercury*, the reason they give is because *Mercury* is conjoined in same particular operations of the brain, and this plant is of known virtue to comfort the brain. But by my rules and daily experience, I find it to be under the dominion of the *Sun* ; First by reason of its elemental qualities as agreeing with heat and dryness : Secondly in regard of its virtues, for all herbs and plants, which are of sweet smell, and are of approved virtues to comfort the heart, brain, nerves and arteries, and vital spirits, as this plant is justly and rationally accounted to be under the dominion of the *Sun* who is the fountain of life, Lord of *Leo* and exalted in *Aries*, whereas *Mercury* has only predominance over some particular operations of the brain, as he has in all the five senses. It's generally approved of all Authors that the bulk of the brain in all creatures, is under the dominion of the *Moon*. The vital and quickening part under the *Sun*, the operation of *Mercury* as aforesaid. Now to gather this plant at the right planetary hour, that so you may have the influence of both planets in question, you must do as before expressed, let those planets concerned be in either *Conjunction*, *Trine*, or *Sextile*, aspect to each other, at the time of gathering, or otherwise let the Moon be separating and applying from the one planet to the other at the time of gathering by any of the before going aspects : *Example*, If I were minded to gather the said sweet marjoram in *September*, 1669, about which time such like plants are in their prime to gather. In which month upon the fourteenth day the *Sun* and *Mercury* are in partile *Conjunction*, but their influence holds above a week before and after, for until they are separated ten degrees from each other their Orbs, Rays, or Influence holds strong to perfection, wherefore you may gather this plant aright upon *Sunday* the fifth day, or upon *Sunday* the tenth day or upon *Sunday* the fifteenth day from the *Sun's*, rising until the *Sun* is about an hour in height ; and likewise in the afternoon between one and two o' clock as appears in the perpetual Almanack for the day appointed. Also you may gather any day of those weeks, when the *Sun* is Lord of the hour, and if the *Moon* be in friendly aspect it's the better ; how to find the Lord of the hour, I have shown elsewhere at the beginning of the second book.

NOTE, That in gathering all kinds of herbs and plants whatsoever, more especially, when you intend to do any great cure, you must get the influential virtue of one of the fortunes, *viz.* the *Sun*, *Jupiter*, or *Venus* to be joined or be in some friendly aspect with that planet, which owns the plant having regard to the infirmity or grief which either by sympathy or antipathy has any relation to the fortune, as instance endive, which is cold and dry under *Mercury* yet in regard it's approved good to cool the heat of the liver, which is under *Jupiter*, therefore let *Jupiter* be in *Conjunction*, *Trine*, or *Sextile* aspect to *Mercury* or the *Moon* separating and applying by any of those aspects from the one planet to the other, when you gather the plant, this is to be done, when an Infortune owns the plant or herb you are minded to gather.

A Plain and Easy way how to gather herbs or plants aright that so you may have the benefit both of the day and hour, when each planet reigns, which owns the plant throughout the year : And will generally serve to gather any Herbs or plants aright for the use of physick, Being fitted for every ten days of the Month throughout the year and so for ever.

NOTE,

All Herbs and Plants, which are under the dominion of the *Sun* are gathered on Sundays : and all those herbs and plants which are under the dominion of the *Moon* are gathered on Mondays : and all those under *Mars* on Tuesdays : and all those under *Mercury* on Wednesdays : and all those under *Jupiter* on Thursdays : and all those under *Venus* on Fridays : and all those under *Saturn* on Saturdays. Now every planet which is Lord of the day, rules the first and the eighth hour of the day, each day being divided into twelve equal parts, which we call the planetary hours (and so the planetary hours are near twice so long in the highest of Summer, as they are in the midst of winter). *Example,* Suppose I were minded to gather herbs or plants under the dominion of *Sol* upon one of the first ten days of *January.* Then upon Sunday from the *Sun's* rising, which is six minutes after eight o'clock until 46 min. past eight in the morning, and likewise from 40 minutes past noon until 20 minutes past one, you may gather any herb or plant under the dominion of the Sun by which account you have the benefit both of the day and hour as aforesaid as appears in the Table following, you may do the like for any other plant or herb whatsoever, always remembering that the planet which is Lord of the day ever rules the first and the eighth hour, divided as aforesaid into twelve equal parts.

		Length of the planetary hours	
	January *the first* 10 *days.*		
Bef. noon	From the Sun's rising which is 6 min after 8 until 46 min. past 8.	h. 0	m. 40
Aft. noon	From 40 min. past noon until 20 min. past 1.		
	January *from the* 10 *day to the* 20 *day.*		
Bef. noon	From the Sun's rising being 47 min. after 7 until 30 min. past 8.	h. 0	m. 43
Aft. noon	From 43 min. past noon until 20 min. past 1.		
	January *from the* 20 *to the end.*		
Bef. noon	From the Sun's rising being 26 min. past 7 until 30 min after 8	h. 0	m. 46
Aft. noon	From 43 min. past noon until 26 min. past 1.		
	February *the first* 10 *days.*		
Bef. noon	From the Sun's rising being 12 min. after 7 until 8 o'clock.	h. 0	m. 48
Aft. noon	From 48 min. past noon until 36 min. past 1.		
	February *from the* 10 *day to the* 20 *day.*		
Bef. noon	From the Sun's rising being 57 mi. past 6 until 40 min. past 7.	h. 0	m. 51
Aft. noon	From 51 min. past noon until 14 min. past 1.		
	February *from the* 20 *day to the end.*		
Bef. noon	From the Sun's rising being 36 min. past 6 until 28 min. past 7.	h. 0	m. 54
Aft. noon	From 54 min. past noon until 48 min. past 1.		

Perpetual Almanack : *LMT, Julian dates*

		Length of the planetary hours
	March *the first* 10 *days.*	
Bef. noon	From the Sun's rising being 7 min. past 6 until 5 min. past 7.	h. m. 0 58
Aft. noon	From 58 min. past noon until 58 min. past 1.	
	March *from the* 10 *day to the* 20 *day.*	
Bef. noon	From the Sun's rising being 6 o'clock until 7 o'clock.	h. m. 1 0
Aft. noon	From one o'clock until 2 o'clock.	
	March *from the* 20 *day the mon. end.*	
Bef. noon	From the Sun's rising being 28 min. after 5 until 33 min. past 6.	h. m. 1 5
Aft .noon	From 5 min. past 1 until 11 min. past two.	
	April *the first* 10 *days.*	
Bef. noon	From the Sun's rising being 3 min. after 5 until 13 min. past 6.	h. m. 1 13
Aft. noon	From 10 min. after 1 until 19 min. past 2.	
	April *from the* 10 *day to the* 20 *day*	
Bef. noon	From the Sun's rising being 45 min. past 4 until 58 min. past 5.	h. m. 1 13
Aft. noon	From 13 min. past 1 until 25 min. past 2.	
	April *from the* 20 *day to the end.*	
Bef. noon	From the Sun's rising being 8 min after 4 until 48 min. past 5:	h. m. 1 14
Aft. noon	From 14 min. past 1 until 29 min. past 2	

		Length of the planetary hours	
	May *the first* 10 *days.*		
Bef. noon	From the Sun's rising being 8 min. after 4 until 37 min. past 5.	h. 1	m. 19
Aft. noon	From 19 min. past 1 until 37 m. past 2.		
	May *from the* 10 *day to the* 20 *day.*		
Bef. noon	From the Sun's rising being 56 min. after 3 until 17 Min. past 5.	h. 1	m. 22
Aft. noon	From 22 min. after 1 until 42 min. past 2.		
	May *from the* 20 *day to the end.*		
Bef. noon	From the Sun's rising being 45 min. after 3 until 8 Min past 5.	h. 1	m. 23
Aft. noon	From 23 min past 1 until 45 m. past 2.		
	June *the first* 10 *days.*		
Bef. noon	From the Sun's rising being 39 min. after 3 until 3 min. past 5.	h. 1	m. 24
Aft. noon	From 24 min. past 1 until 47 min. past 2.		
	June *from the* 10 *to the* 20 *day.*		
Bef. noon	From the Sun's rising being 39 min. after 3 until 3 min. past 5.	h. 1	m. 24
Aft. noon	From 24 min. past 1 until 47 min. past 2		
	June *the* 20 *to the end.*		
Bef. noon	From the Sun's rising being 44 min. past 3 until 7 min. past 5.	h. 1	m. 23
Aft. noon	From 23 min. past 1 until 46 min. past 2.		

Perpetual Almanack : *LMT, Julian dates*

		Length of the planetary hours

July *the first* 10 *days*.

		h.	m.
Bef. noon	From the Sun's rising being 35 min. after 3 until 16 min. after 5. }	1	22
Aft. noon	From 21 min. past 1 until 42 min. past 2.		

July *from the* 10 *day to the* 20 *day*.

		h.	m.
Bef. noon	From the Sun's rising being 8 min. past 4 until 27 min. past 5. }	1	19
Aft. noon	From 19 min. past 1 until 37 min. past 2		

July *from the* 20 *day to the end*.

		h.	m.
Bef. noon	From the Sun's rising being 26 min. past 4 until 49 min. past 5. }	1	16
Aft. noon	From 16 min. past 1 until 22 min. past 2.		

August *the first* 10 *days*.

		h.	m.
Bef. noon	From the Sun's rising being 45 min. past 4 until 58 min. past 5. }	1	13
Aft. noon	From 13 min. past 1 until 25 min. past 2.		

August *from the* 10 *day to the* 20 *day*.

		h.	m.
Bef. noon	From the Sun's rising being 3 min. after 5 until 13 min past 6. }	1	10
Aft. noon	From 6 min. past 1 until 13 min. past 2.		

August *from the* 20 *day to the end*.

		h.	m.
Bef. noon	From the Sun's rising being 23 min. after 5 until 47 min. past 6. }	1	6
Aft. noon	From 6 min. past 1 until 13 min. past two.		

		Length of the planetary hours	

September the first 10 days.

		h.	m.
Bef. noon	From the Sun's rising being 47 min. after 5 until 47 min. past 6.	1	2
Aft. noon	From 2 min. after 1 until 4 min. past 2.		

September from the 10 day to the 20 day.

		h.	m.
Bef. noon	From the Sun's rising being 6 min. past 6 until 5 min. past 7.	0	59
Aft. noon	From 59 min. after noon until 58 min. past 1.		

September from the 20 day to the end.

		h.	m.
Bef. noon	From the Sun's rising being 26 m. after 6 until 22 min. past 7	0	56
Aft. noon	From 56 min. after noon until 50 min. past 1.		

October the first 10 days.

		h.	m.
Bef. noon	From the Sun's rising being 50 min. after 6 until 42 min. past 7.	0	52
Aft. noon	From 52 min. after noon until 43 min. past 1.		

October from the 10 day to the 20 day.

		h.	m.
Bef. noon	From the Sun's rising being 11 min. after 7 until 8 o'clock.	0	49
Aft. noon	From 49 min. past noon until 37 min. past 1.		

October from the 20 day to the end.

		h.	m.
Bef. noon	From the Sun's rising being 27 min. past 7 until 4 min. past 8.	0	4 6
Aft. noon	From 46 min. past noon until 31 min. past 1.		

		Length of the planetary hours	
	November *the first* 10 *days.*		
Bef. noon	From the Sun's rising being 48 min. after 7 until 30 min. past 8.	h. 0	m. 43
Aft. noon	From 43 min. past noon, until 24 min. past 1.		
	Nov. *from the* 10 *day to the* 20 *day.*		
Bef. noon	From the Sun's rising being 3 min. after 8 until 43 min. past 8.	h. 0	m. 40
Aft. noon	From 40 min. past noon until 19 min. past 1.		
	November *from the* 20 *day to the end.*		
Bef. noon	From the Sun's rising being 45 min. past 8 until 53 min after 8	h. 0	m. 38
Aft. noon	From 38 min. past noon until 15 min. past 1.		
	December *the first* 10 *days.*		
Bef. noon	From the Sun's rising being 20 min. after 8 until 57 min. past 8.	h. 0	m. 37
Aft. noon	From 37 min. past noon until 14 min. past 1.		
	December *from the* 10 *day to the* 20 *day.*		
Bef. noon	From the Sun's rising being 20 min. past 8 until 57 min past 8.	h. 0	m. 37
Aft. noon	From 37 min. past noon until 14 min. past 1.		
	December *from the* 20 *day to the end.*		
Bef. noon	From the Sun's rising being 15 min. past 8 until 53 min. past 8.	h. 0	m. 38
Aft. noon	From 38 min. past noon until 15 min. past 1.		

Concerning Numbers attributed to the seven Planets with the Reasons thereof, agreeing with Cornelius Agrippa, an excellent Philosopher, besides my own daily practice and experience.

Saturn.

Numbers attributed to the planet.

TO this Planet *Saturn* belongs three numbers, *viz.* two seven, nine. The number two as being next beneath the starry firmament ; and also as being one of the two infortunes, the number seven, as being the seventh in order, and highest from the earth. Its also a number fatal and climacterical as joined with the number nine. Also the number nine is a number fatal and climacterical as joined with the number seven : For nine times 7 makes 63, which number all philosophers hold to be fatal and climacterical by reason the nines and the sevens meet.

2

7

9

Jupiter

Jupiter has three numbers, allotted to him, *viz*, one, three eight ; The number one, as being the head and chief fortunes ; the number three, as being the third star or planet in order from the starry firmament beneath *Saturn* also, as being one of the three fortunes. The number eight as containing the mystery of Justice and Religion : for Jupiter in astrology always represents the sober Priest or Minister, according to which number Christ was circumcised : also we read of eight degrees of blessedness, &c.

1

3

8

Mars

Mars has four numbers allotted to him, *viz.* two, four, seven, nine : The number two, as being one of the two infortunes : The number four, as being the fourth in number from the starry firmament next to Jupiter : The number seven as being a number fatal and climacterical as joined with nine : Also he has the number nine as being a number fatal and climacterical, as joined with seven. This planet as likewise *Saturn* are both enemies to Nature.

Numbers attributed to the planet.

2
4
7
9

Sol.

The **Sun** has five several numbers allotted to him, *viz.* one, three, four, seven, ten, twelve. The number one as being sole Monarch of the heavens : The number three as being one of the three fortunes : The number four, from the four quarters of the year : The number ten as being the number of the end of life, as multiplied by seven : The number twelve as passing through the twelve signs of the Zodiac.

1
3
4
10
12

Venus.

Venus has three numbers allotted to her, *viz.* two, three, nine : The number two as being female. The number three as being one of the three fortunes : The number six as being the number of generation consisting of two threes.

2
3
6

Mercury.

Numbers attributed to the planet.

This Planet **Mercury** has two numbers allotted to him, *viz.* two five : The number two, as being part male and part female. And therefore called the hermaphrodite. The number five as having predominancy over the operation of the five senses.

2
5

Moon.

The **Moon** has three numbers allotted to her, *viz.* two six, nine : The number two as being female : The number six as being the number of generation : The number nine, as being the utmost receptacle of all celestial influences.

2
6
9

The Astrological way, whereby to discover all kinds of Diseases, or Infirmities incident to the body of Man : And likewise how to know whether the Sick shall live or die : also the time, when either Recovery or Death may be expected ; with the true Astrological way of curing each Disease which is curable, as follows.

IN the first place, before we come to set forth the Method of cure, it will be necessary to find what the grief is, and from what cause ; without which its impossible to do any great cures. There are two ways by which Judgment may be given herein : The one Astrologically by a Figure of twelve Houses, which is accounted to be the most assured and exactest way : the other is by the Moon according as she is afflicted by the malevolent Planets, having regard to the signs or constellations, wherein she was afflicted, at the time of decumbiture : This way may serve generally in acute diseases, and I find by my daily practice, that one shall seldom err herein, but in case of such Diseases, which are natural from the birth, or have been of very long standing, or more especially, if there be any suspicion of Witchcraft, a Figure of twelve houses is most rational. I shall briefly show the way of both : But in regard a Figure of twelve Houses and the astrological way in giving judgement thereupon may seem difficult at the first, especially to those, who have never formerly read or studied any whit in this Science : And further considering that many, who are well willers hereunto either may want time, or be unwilling to take the pains herein, may neglect the study hereof, and so this my writing may prove useless to them, I have for the satisfaction and encouragement of all well-willers to this study and practice of Physick, set forth one general way in giving judgment, either by the Moon afflicted in acute diseases, which terminate in a month, or by the Sun in Chronic diseases, which are of above a month's standing : This being the very way of my own daily practice and experience for many years, wherein you shall seldom or never fail, especially in acute diseases, as for other Chronic and long lasting griefs there will be more time allotted to consider of them : The truth is long continued infirmities (and some others) require more inspection than that only of the *Sun* and *Moon* afflicted and therefore a figure of twelve houses will be proper to give judgement therein for many times the ascendant, sixth and twelfth houses with their Lords will be concerned therein, as shall be shown in order. Also it will be necessary after the grief is known, to know the critical, intercidental, and judicial days and times ; being the times for change either of life or death, which is done by a critical figure divided into 16 equal parts, as shall be shown in the next paper.

The way to find the disease by the Sun and Moon afflicted.

In the first place by an Almanack take notice, what sign the *Moon* is in, when the Sick first takes their bed, and by what planet or planets she is afflicted, whether of *Saturn* or *Mars* (or *Mercury*, which is much of the nature of Saturn). Then having recourse to the rules elsewhere in this Book under the titles of the *Moon* by *Saturn* or *Mars* afflicted ; there you shall find the disease and the cause thereof. The Almanack, which you use herein must be such a one which sets forth the daily motions of the planets : I shall give one or two examples hereof, as follows, A Friend of mine took his bed the 10th day of *October* 1667 at a quarter past one o'clock after noon, the *Moon* being of nine degrees in *Sagittarius* and *Mars* in eight degrees thirty five minutes in *Virgo*, which argues that *Mars* is in platic square to the *Moon*, we call that a platic aspect, which does not perfectly accord in degrees and minutes, and if *Mars* had been but one degree in *Virgo*, yet we should account it a platic Square, by reason that the Orbs, Rays, or Influence of the *Moon* to any planet begin to operate, when she is within ten degrees aspecting any planet (as is shown at large elsewhere). Now to find the Grief with its cause, you must repair to the place in this book entitled, The Moon in Sagittarius of Mars oppressed, as in page 65 which shows that the Sick is tormented with a strong fever and choleric passions, &c. occasioned by surfeiting or too much repletion as there more at large appears : the next thing to consider is to know whether the Sick shall live or die, and the time when either death or recovery may be expected : Now in regard that the *Moon* is applying by a friendly Sextile aspect to *Venus* a fortune, and free from combustion and not in that part of the Zodiac called *via combusta* (as shall be shown more at large elsewhere) I concluded that the sick would recover (and so he did) ; had the *Moon* applied to the infortunes ♄ or ♂ and no fortune interposed his friendly Rays, then I should have concluded that the sick would have died of this sickness, to know when the time of recovery will be is found by a critical figure or circle divided into 16 equal parts, I shall not stand or spend time to give you the definition of each term of art ; Only thus much I say, the intercidental time or divident part of the circle is not so dangerous ; as the judicial time or part, nor yet the judicial time so dangerous as the critical time.

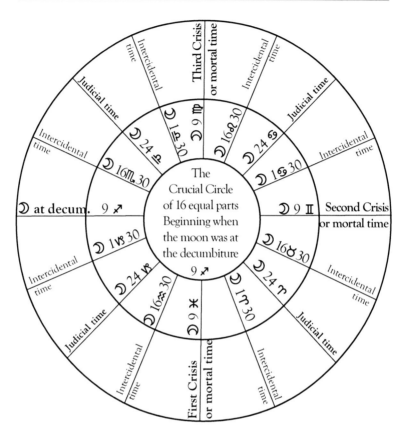

Note, That in this critical figure each part contains 22 *deg.* 30 *min.* you must begin where the *Moon* was at the decumbiture, *viz.* in 9 *deg.* ♐ to which you must add 22 *deg.* 30 min. Now in regard there is 30 *deg.* in every sign you must set down 1 *deg.* 30 *Capricorn* for the first intercidental time, to which 1 *deg.* 30 *min.* you must add 22 *deg.* 30 *min.* which makes 24 *Capricorn*, for the first judicial time : Now if you add 22 *deg.* 30 *min.* to the last number it makes 16 *deg.* 30 *min. Aquarius*, which is the second intercidental time, and if you add 22 *deg.* 30 *min.* to the last number , it makes 9 *deg. Pisces*, which is the first crisis or mortal time, according to which account you must go round the circle, as appears by the figure, now to know when the time of recovery will be you must observe by a critical figure, when the Moon upon a critical day meets with any friendly aspect of either of the fortunes, *viz. Jupiter* or *Venus* or *Sol* or *Leo*, for then the time of recovery may be expected. This critical figure being set for a friend of mine at the time aforesaid. I observed each change, and alteration of his distemper ; and I always found that upon the critical and judicial days and times, he was ever most afflicted. The reason is because the *Quartiles*, *Oppositions*, and *Semi-quartile* aspects are more pernicious and hateful aspects, than any other, as the intercidental times, which happen between the critical and judicial times consisting only of 22 *deg.* and a half, which we call a *Semi Semi Quartile* aspect, they seldom prove mortal, by reason the aspect is not so bad and forcible as the other, it being but half the half quartile aspect, yet notwithstanding sometimes in perperacute mortal sicknesses. I have known the Sick depart, when the Moon came to a partile evil aspect of the infortunes, no fortune interposing their friendly rays upon an intercidental time, but this is not usual ; but as concerning the time of recovery of my Friend before mentioned it was upon the fourth and last critical day, the Moon being returned to the place she was in at the decumbiture : at which time she applied to the *Sextile* of *Venus* and *Trine* of *Jupiter*, which happened upon the sixth day of *November* after midnight, would my friend have been let blood, he might questionless have recovered upon the second crisis, at what time the Moon applied to the *Trine* of *Venus*, now had this Sickness continued longer, then we account the grief Chronic, and then we give judgement by the Sun afflicted, as before we did by the Moon. But all acute griefs end usually before the Moon goes round the *Zodiac* ; some griefs are peracute and those end sooner, others are perperacute, and those commonly make a quick dispatch one way or other. But of this I have treated more at large elsewhere.

Judgment upon an Imaginary decumbiture,

For the better explanation hereof I shall instance two or three Imaginary Decumbitures as follows. Suppose one should take his Bed *April* the 10th 1668 at Noon, the *Moon* being then in 12 *deg.* 50 *min.* in the Sign *Leo* and *Saturn*, in 12 *deg.* 50 *min.* in the Sign *Aquarius*, now this is called a partile opposition aspect, by reason the *Moon* and *Saturn* are just in the same *deg.* and *min.* opposite to each other: had the Sick took his bed 16 hours sooner, or later, then it would have been called a Platic opposition, for as I have said elsewhere, the influence of the *Moon* and Planets begins to appear when she is 10 *deg.* distant from any aspect which will take up near 20 *hours* motion before and after separation ; Now to know what the Grief is, you must seek out the place in this Book entitled the *Moon* in *Leo* of *Saturn* oppressed, which argues the Sick shall be troubled with unkindly heat in the Breast, and a violent Fever, with faintness at the heart, or swounding fits, and inclining to the Black jaundies occasioned from ill Melancholy blood, &c. Now to know whether the Sick shall live or die, and the time when either recovery, or Death may be expected, is as follows.

First the *Moon* is increasing in light. Secondly she is not in that place in the Zodiac called *via combusta*, which is from the middle of the Sign *Libra* to the middle of *Scorpio*. Thirdly the *Moon* separates from *Jupiter*, a fortune, and applies to a friendly Trine aspect of the *Sun*, fountain of life. Fourthly, the *Moon* is free from combustion of the *Sun*. A Planet is under combustion when he is not fully elongated 7 *deg.* 30 *min.* from him. We have only two Testimonies of Death, which is first, *Saturn* being in opposition of the *Moon* at the time of decumbiture. Secondly his being more strong than the *Moon*, yet commonly a Planet strong is not so malicious as those which are weak and peregrine; however it appears that there are four testimonies of Life and but two of Death, wherefore we may conclude according to the Rules of Art that the Sick shall recover: Now to know the time when, you must by a Critical figure of 16 equal parts, take notice when the *Moon* upon any Intercidental, Judicial or Critical day meets with any benevolent aspect of the fortunes, be it *Sun, Jupiter, Venus,* or *Dragons head,* no evil Planet interposing their bad Influence for then the Sick shall recover, which according to the Critical figure will be upon the 12th day of *April* about one o'clock at night, at which time the *Moon* will be in 14 *deg.* of the Sign *Virgo* and *Jupiter* in 14 *deg.* of *Taurus* making a partile *Trine* to each other, but the Sick shall begin to recover sooner at the first intercidental time, which is about six o'clock in the morning (at which time the *Moon* will be 5 *deg.* 10 *min.* in *Virgo,* which is 22 *deg.* 30 *min.* distant from the place she was in at the decumbiture) for as I have already declared the influence of the *Moon* begins to operate, when she is ten degrees distant from any aspect of the planets.

Concerning Acute Griefs.

Note, That at the time of decumbiture of any sick person, if the *Moon* be free from the bad aspects of the infortunes, which are *Saturn, Mars, Mercury,* or *Dragons* tail that then (more especially) if the fortunes *Jupiter* or *Venus* attend upon the next judicial or critical day or time that the *Moon* meets with any friendly aspect of the fortunes, no ill planet opposing, the Sick shall recover: but commonly acute griefs are seldom ended before the first critical time, at which time the *Moon* makes a *Quartile* aspect to the place she was in at the decumbiture, consisting of 90 *deg.* The *Moon* always goes this 90 *deg.* or fourth part of the Zodiac in less than eight days; sometimes acute griefs last until the *Moon* has passed over three critical days or times, *Viz.* until she returns to the place she was in at the decumbiture making the fourth crisis ; An Example hereof is of my friend before mentioned : and if by the Rules aforesaid you find that the grief is mortal, then you must proceed forward round the critical figure, until you find the mortal time, according to the rules before mentioned, and you must do the like upon the rules for the time of recovery.

Concerning Peracute griefs.

There are also some Infirmities and Sicknesses which end usually before the first judicial time is over (called peracute griefs) at which time the *Moon* makes a *Semi-quartile* aspect to the place she was in at the decumbiture, consisting of 45 *deg.* now this aspect is not so pernicious as the *Quartile,* yet oftentimes the Sick die before this aspect is over ; more especially when the *Moon* at that time meets with the infortunes, and no fortune interposing their friendly rays. This *Semi-Quartile* aspect or judicial time, the *Moon* finishes in less than four days likewise on the contrary by the rules aforesaid the Sick may recover at the said judicial time.

Concerning Perperacute Sicknesses.

There are also some Sicknesses perperacute, and such griefs commonly terminate before the first intercidental time is over at which time the *Moon* makes a *Semi-Semi-Quartile* aspect to the place she was in at the decumbiture, which consists of 22 *deg.* 30 *min.* containing the 16th part of the critical figure, more especially when the infortunes afflict the *Moon,* at that time no fortune attending : It was observed, that in the time of the plague, that many thousands died before the first intercidental time was over, which number or time the *Moon* finishes in less than two days. And many lived not one day,

Another Judgement Upon a Decumbiture   35

dying immediately so soon as they were struck, which we call the time of decumbiture or first mortal time. I have known the like both in Apoplexies and Convulsions, mother fits, and risings in the throat, and such like griefs.

Another Judgement given upon a decumbiture Figure.

I shall take an imaginary time, and so give judgement thereupon for the better informing of young Students herein. I could have inserted many exemplary figures of my own, but considering that new Almanacks may be had when happily old ones may be lost I therefore thought this way most profitable to instruct the learner. I shall instance the 2nd day of *April* 1668 about nine o'clock at night, at which time I will suppose one took his bed : Now the question is what the grief is, and whether the Sick will live or die : And when either death or recovery may be expected, you must in the first place by an Almanack find in what sign the *Moon* is, and how aspected : Now at the hour and time aforesaid, the *Moon* will be in 5 *deg.* 48 *min.* of the sign *Aquarius*, and at the same time I find *Mars* to be in 5 *deg.* 48 *min.* of the sign *Scorpio*, which makes a partile *Square* aspect consisting of 90 *deg.* : Now to find what the grief is you must repair to the place in this book, where it is written, *The Moon in* Aquarius *of* Mars *oppressed*, which argues, that the Sick shall be troubled with great pain at the heart and with swooning fits also very feverish, likewise a pain in the breast with difficulty of breathing, and the blood swelling in all the veins, the cause of this sickness proceeding from violent affections and vehement passions, &c. Now the next thing to consider is to know whether the Sick be like to live or die ; and the time when either death or recovery may be expected. First the *Moon* is decreasing in light, Secondly the *Moon* departs from the *Square* of *Mars* and applies to the *Conjunction* of *Saturn* both inimical planets : Thirdly, neither *Sol, Jupiter,* or *Venus* cast their friendly rays or influence at the time aforesaid to the *Moon,* wherefore according to the rules aforesaid, the sick person will die : To find the time, when you must frame a critical figure of sixteen equal parts as aforesaid, beginning at the place where the *Moon* was at the decumbiture, making that the first critical or mortal time, which if the Sick escape, then at the next critical or mortal time, you must observe how the *Moon* is aspected, at which time you shall find the *Moon* meets with the opposition of ♂ being upon the 29th day of *April* in the Month aforesaid at one o'clock after noon : Now in regard there is no fortunate planet interposing their friendly rays at that time we may conclude that the sick will depart, and not before, because the *Sun* at intercidental and judicial times meets with no bad aspect of the infortunes. Yet notwithstanding I have known some, who have been mortally struck according to any rational man's judgment at the decumbiture in acute griefs, who through God's blessing, having an expert and skillful Physician, and having withstood the bad influence of the afflicting planets, at the first mortal time beyond expectation, upon the next critical time have recovered, and so it may happily prove to some, who shall take their bed at the time aforesaid. The reason is because between the time of decumbiture and first crisis, there is usually near seven days time, during which time (special remedies being applied) the Sick may happily be the better enabled to withstand the encounter, more especially if the intercidental and judicial times be freed from the evil aspects of the infortunes, as here it falls out at this last decumbiture. The truth is life and death is in the hands of God, and whatsoever stars foreshow, yet he by his power and blessing upon the means used can preserve life, when he pleases, wherefore the sick ought not at any time to despair. For I myself have often times recovered my Patient having out lived the first mortal time as aforesaid, but I must needs say such changes and chances are seldom seen, for where one escapes many die for the stars are God's Messengers, and what they foreshow, does assuredly without miracle come to pass. Concerning the way and manner how to cure each distemper, I have shown elsewhere.

Concerning the Astrological way of giving Judgement by a Sign of 12 Houses.

Although what is already written, I have known by good experience to hold true by many examples it being for the most part the method of my daily practice ; yet for the benefit and better satisfaction of Practitioners, and others, well-willers thereunto, especially such who desire further inspection into this Art, I shall in the next place show how in an Astrological way judgement may be given by a figure of 12 Houses. For I must confess that in such infirmities, which are natural from the birth, and likewise some chronic griefs, which have been of long continuance, and likewise such infirmities, wherein there is any suspicion of witchcraft, cannot so exactly be discovered by the *Sun* or *Moon* afflicted, as by a sign of twelve houses for the ascendant, sixth, eighth, and twelfth Houses with their Lords will be for the most part concerned therein as shall be shown in order as follows. In the first place you must erect your figure : either for the time of decumbiture, or for the time of any strong fit (if any be) or upon the receipt of the Urine, or time of the first visitation of the Patient, and you must be sure for to frame, and vary your ascendant, that it together with its Lord may exactly personate the Sick. Secondly you must in order set down the Cusp of every House. Thirdly you must set down the Characters of the Planets in every House, which for to do, and likewise how to frame the ascendant, I shall briefly declare. But before you can proceed herein, you must perfectly know the Characters of the seven Planets and twelve signs, and the five Aspects of the Planets; and the Houses of each Planet.

The Characters of the Seven Planets with the Dragons Head and Tail

♄ Saturn } ♂ Mars   } ♀ Venus   } ☽ Luna } ☊ Dragons Head
♃ Jupiter } ☉ Sun   } ☿ Mercury }   } ☋ Dragons Tail

The Characters of the twelve Signs, with the parts of the Body by them signified; And how they stand opposite to each other in the Zodiac, as follows.

♈ *Aries* Head and Face.   ♎ *Libra* Reins and Loins.
♉ *Taurus* Neck and Throat.   ♏ *Scorpio* Secrets and Bladder.
♊ *Gemini* Arms & Shoulders.   ♐ *Sagittarius* The Thighs.
♋ *Cancer* Breast, Stom. & Ribs.   ♑ *Capricorn* The Knees.
♌ *Leo* Heart and Back.   ♒ *Aquarius* The Legs.
♍ *Virgo* Bowels and Guts.   ♓ *Pisces* The Feet.

The five Aspects of the Planets.

☌ *Conjunction,* That is when any two Planets are in one and the same degree of any Sign.

✶ *Sextile,* That is when any two Planets are 60 degrees from each other : And contains a sixth part of the Zodiac.

☐ *Square,* That is when any two Planets are 90 degrees from each other : And contains a fourth part of the Zodiac.

△ *Trine,* That is when any two Planets are 120 degrees from each other : And contains a third part of the Zodiac.

☍ *Opposition,* That is when any two Planets are 180 degrees from each other : And contains half the Zodiac.

What Every House Concerns in Decumbiture

NOTE, That there is 30 *deg*. in every Sign, and two Signs make a sextile aspect, three Signs make a square, four signs make a Trine, six Signs make an Opposition, which contains half the Zodiac. The whole contains 360 *deg*, which is 12 times 30 *deg*.

The Houses of the Planets

♄ *Saturn* has two houses; *viz*. The signs ♑ *Capricorn*, and ♒ *Aquarius* : ♃ *Jupiter* has two Houses ♐ *Sagittarius*, and ♓ *Pisces* : ♂ *Mars* has two Houses ♈ *Aries*, and ♏ *Scorpio* : ☉ *Sol*, has but one House, which is ♌ *Leo* : ♀ *Venus* has two Houses ♎ *Libra* and ♉ *Taurus* : *Mercury* has two Houses ♊ *Gemini* and ♍ *Virgo*, ☽ the *Moon* has but one House, which is ♋ *Cancer*.

How to Frame the twelve Houses, and what every House concerns, in a Decumbiture Figure.

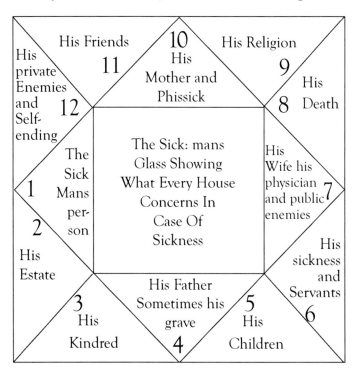

THE next thing to consider is, to have knowledge how to insert the twelve Signs upon the cusp of every House, and likewise to set the seven Planets in those Signs : But before we can proceed therein it will be necessary to understand the use of an Ephemeris or Almanack, which sets forth the daily motions of the planets. And for the better informing of young Students herein, I shall for example set down in order for the month of *October,* 1667 the form as usually is printed, and show the use thereof until the tenth day of the said month ; which will be enough whereby to understand, not only the residue of that month, but also every other month throughout the year, provided always that your Almanack must be such a one which sets forth the daily motions of the planets, whose Title page to every month is as follows,

		\multicolumn{8}{c}{*October* has XXXI days}

Month days	Week days	\multicolumn{8}{c}{The daily motions of the Planets and ☊}
		♄	♃R	♂	☉	♀	☿	☽	☊
		♑	♉	♍	♎	♎	♎	♌	♊
1	a	25 35	1 59	3 8	18 2	7 21	3 25	1 48	10 29
2	b	25 36	1 51	3 45	19 1	8 36	5 9	14 25	10 26
3	c	25 37	1 43	4 21	20 1	9 51	6 45	27 25	10 23
4	d	25 39	1 35	4 57	21 1	11 6	8 25	10♍ 16	10 20
5	e	25 40	1 27	5 33	22 0	12 2	10 6	24 48	10 17
6	F	25 42	1 19	6 14	23 0	13 37	11 47	8 ♎ 18	10 14
7	g	25 43	1 11	6 48	24 0	14 52	13 28	21 47	10 11
8	a	25 45	1 3	7 23	25 0	16 7	15 9	6 ♏ 18	10 8
9	b	25 47	0 55	7 59	26 0	17 22	16 50	23 39	10 4
10	c	25 49	0 47	8 35	27 0	18 38	18 32	8 ♐ 31	10 1

Concerning the use of the Ephemeris.

The first column on the left shows the days of the month, the second column shows the week days, the next column shows the daily motion of *Saturn*, the sign next beneath his character shows what sign he is in and the numbers next beneath that shows how far *Saturn* is entered into the sign for every day, the first number is for degrees, the second minutes, and so forwards for every planet accordingly. *Example,* ♄ *Saturn* the first day is 25 *deg.* 35 *min.* in the sign *Capricorn* : the second day he is 25 *deg.* 36 *min.* in *Capricorn* : the third day he is 25 *deg.* 37 *min.* in *Capricorn* : the fourth day he is 25 *deg.* 39 *min.* in *Capricorn* and so forward. In the next column is ♃ *Jupiter* and the sign ♉ *Taurus* beneath which argues that ♃ *Jupiter* is in the sign ♉ *Taurus*, and over against the first day is the numbers 1 *deg.* 59 *min.* which shows that he is so far in the sign : the second day is but 1 *deg.* 51 *min.* the third day he is 1 *deg.* 43 *min.* the fourth day he is 1 *deg.* 35 *min.* and so onward, this planet's numbers decrease daily by reason he is retrograde and moves backward, as sometimes all the rest will, except the Sun and Moon. In the next Column is ♂ *Mars* and underneath the sign *Virgo*, and under that the numbers 3 *deg.* 8 *min.* which argues that Mars the first day is gotten so far in the sign *Virgo*, the second day he is 3 *deg.* 45 *min.* in the sign *Virgo*, the third day 4 *deg.* 21 *min.* The fourth day he is 4 *deg.* 57 *min* in *Virgo*, and so downward as you find in the Table ; you may do the like for the rest of the planets accordingly.

How to erect a Scheme or Figure according to any time given

The usual time whereby to erect a Figure concerning any Patient, is first by the time of falling ill, or most properly, when the patients first betake them to their bed, which we call the time of decumbiture : But if that may not be had, as sometimes 'twill fall out, especially in Chronic griefs, then you must take the time, when the urine is first brought, or the time of any strong fit, if any be. Or the time when you first visit the patient, provided always that you so vary your ascendant, that it together with its Lord may exactly personate the sick, without which no true judgment can be given, by reason the Ascendant, fourth, sixth, eighth, and twelfth Houses are concerned, now if you fail in the first, there can be no certainty in the rest, how to know what bodily shape belongs to each Figure, and planet is shown elsewhere in this Book : for the better understanding hereof I shall insert one example as follows, A friend of mine being very ill took his bed, *October* the 10, 1667, at a quarter past one o'clock in the afternoon, according to which time I erected a figure as follows, having by an Almanack found out that page entitled *The daily Motions of the Planets*, as is before expressed for the Month of *October*, you must seek for the 10 day of the said month, and move forward in a straight line, until you come to the sixth column, and under the Characters over head thus expressed there you shall find the number 27, ☉|♎ which shows that the Sun is gotten into the sign *Libra* 27 deg. upon the tenth day aforesaid, with this number 27, you must enter the Table of Houses, which you shall find at the end of the Almanac, and seek out the page, where it is written *Sol* in *Libra*. And in the column under 80 *min*. the signs going down in a straight line, there you shall find time number 17, and in the column next adjoining on the left hand under time title of time from noon moving downward to the same line, where is the number 27 before mentioned, there you shall find the numbers thus printed, *viz*. 13, 40, 12, but the number 12 being but seconds you may leave out and so take only the two first numbers 13, 40, which you must set in some place by itself, then you must add to that number the time of the day, when the sick first took his bed being a quarter past one o'clock afternoon, as for example:

How to Erect a Figure 43

	h.	m.
Time from noon	13	40
The time of the day, when the Sick took his bed	1	15
Note that the 15 *min.* stands for a quarter of an hour, there being 60 in an hour.	14	55

Now had the Sick took his bed at one o'clock at night, then it's called the thirteenth hour, for in Astrology, we begin to count both the days and hours from noon. The numbers before mentioned being added together make 14.55. This number you must find out under the Title of time from noon or the nearest to it being 14.59, which wants but one minute from which sum, or place, you must move forward in the same time, and under every column belonging to each house, you shall find both the sign over head and the number beneath, which is the sign and number you must set down upon the Cusp of every House in the figure as follows:

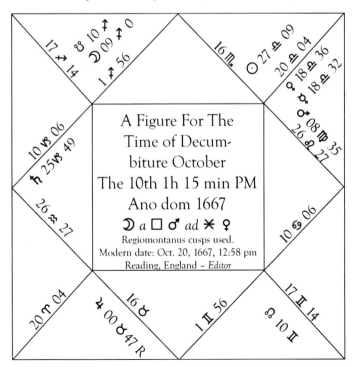

For the cusp of the tenth House *Scorpio* 16. For the eleventh house *Sagitary* 1.56. For the twelfth house *Sagitary* 17.14. For the first house, called the ascendant *Capricorn* 10.6. For the second house *Aquarius* 27.26. For the third house *Aries* 20.4. Now these first six houses being finished, the other six whose signs are opposite are of the same numbers : What signs are opposite to each other I have already declared. *Example* : Over against the sign *Scorpio* 16, being the cusp of the tenth house is *Taurus* 16, the cusp of the fourth house, and over against *Sagitary* 1. 56, being the cusp of the eleventh house, is *Gemini* 1.56 the cusp of the fifth house, and over against *Sagitary* 17.14, the cusp of the twelfth house, is *Gemini* 17.14, the cusp of the sixth house, and over against *Capricorn* 10.6, the cusp of the ascendant, is *Cancer* 10.6, and over against *Aquarius* 27.26, is *Leo* 27.26, and over against *Aries* 20.4, is *Libra* 20.4, as appears by the figure.

The next thing material is to set the planets in those figures, and houses, which for to do you must by the Almanack find out the page before mentioned, for the month of *October*. And from the tenth day moving in a right line, you shall in each column find the numbers of degrees and minutes according as each planet has gotten into each sign : *Example*, The first number is 25 *deg.* 49 *min.* and *Saturn* is over the head of *Capricorn*, which argues that *Saturn* is so many degrees and minutes entered into *Capricorn*, which degrees and minutes you must set in the first house, as by the Figure appears.

In the next column is 0 *deg.* 47 *min.* and *Jupiter* is over the head of *Taurus*, which shows that *Jupiter* is forty seven minutes in *Taurus*, which number with the character of *Jupiter* must be set in the third house.

In the next column is 8 *deg.* 35 *min.* and *Mars* is over the head of *Virgo*, which argues that *Mars* is gotten so far into *Virgo*, and must be set in the eighth house.

In the next column is 27 *deg.* and *Sol* is over the head of *Libra*.

In the next column is 18 *deg.* 38 *min.* and *Venus* is over the head of *Libra*.

In the next column is 18 *deg.* 32 *min.*, and *Mercury* is over the head of *Libra*.

In the next column is 8 *deg.* 31 *min.* and Luna is over the head of *Sagitary*, which argues that the *Moon* was at noon so far entered the Sign *Sagitary*, but in regard it was above an hour after noon when the Sick took his bed, there must be half a degree, which is 30 minutes added to the *Moon's* motion, for by reason of her quick moving, she gets one degree in two hours, wherefore we must set the Moon in nine degrees *Sagitary*; you must do the like in all other figures : Had he took his bed at midnight you must have added six degrees, and then the *Moon* would have been fourteen degrees thirty one minutes entered *Sagitary*. Now having set the signs on the cusps of every house, and the planets in those signs as by the figure appears : I shall in the next place show how to give judgement thereupon, and to thereby discover the grief as follows.

How to give judgement by the Figure of twelve Houses.

THE general way, especially in acute griefs, is to give judgment by the *Moon* being in any of the twelve signs and by the infirmities afflicted, as I have already declared : And this being an acute grief, judgment must be given accordingly, yet notwithstanding I shall by this figure set forth his natural infirmities or griefs, and so instruct the Leaner how to give judgement in any other chronic griefs by the signs on the ascendant, sixth house and their Lords afflicted. For some lasting and obscure griefs cannot be discovered by the *Sun* and *Moon* afflicted. In the first place you must observe whether the ascendant, which is the first house, or the sixth house, or their Lords be any way afflicted by the malevolent planets *Saturn*, *Mars*, *Mercury*, or the *Sun*, for sometimes the *Sun* may and will afflict more, especially if the grief lies about the heart, or in the arteries, or vital spirits. In the next place it will be necessary to know whether the grief be natural, or whether it came by Witchcraft or Sorcery : Now if you find the Lord of the twelfth house in the ascendant or if the Lord of the twelfth being in the sixth, or Lord of the sixth in the twelfth, or if the Lord of the ascendant be combust, that is, when the *Sun* is not above eight degrees thirty minutes distant from him, or if one planet be Lord of the ascendant and twelfth house, and an infortune, then you may conclude that the grief is more than natural, more especially where there is any just suspicion thereof, which may be somewhat deferred by heeding well the nature of their distempers, as I have shown elsewhere : But in this Figure I find no such thing ; wherefore I concluded, the grief was natural ; occasioned by his own disorder of body : as shall be shown in order.

Sometimes I have known the ascendant, the sixth house, or their Lords have been afflicted by the Lord of the twelfth house and yet the sickness was not from Witchcraft, notwithstanding, those suspected evils ; for if *Jupiter* and *Venus*, or the *Sun*, cast their friendly aspects to the afflicted Planet or Cusp of the House aforesaid, that then the grief came by some disorder of body : Also, if that Lord of the ascendant be in the twelfth, or in the sixth, the grief is natural : For from the twelfth house, we give judgment of self-undoing, so well as otherwise ; but any rational experienced practitioner may easily distinguish, the natural diseases, from the unnatural, by heeding well the manner of their distempers, as aforesaid : And generally

How to Give Judgement by the Figure 47

I find that those who are taken in this snare of Witchcraft, that at the time of any strong fit, or when they are more than usually tormented, that then the ascendant together with its Lord exactly personates the sick ; and at that very time, the Lord of the twelfth house does one way or other afflict, either the ascendant, or its Lord ; or that an infortune Lord of the ascendant and twelfth house, which may so happen, when the proper ascendant is intercepted in the first house, as I have often times experimented.

I shall now proceed to give judgment upon the decumbiture figure before mentioned ; and in the first place, describe the person of the sick.

Secondly, By rules discover, whether the sick shall live or die, if live, how long time before recovery.

Thirdly, I shall by rules set forth, what the grief is, and from what case.

Fourthly, How and which way he was recovered.

The man's person is described by the ascendant *Capricorn*, and *Saturn* his being therein who is Lord thereof, *viz*. one of a middle stature, full and well set, of a dark or swarthy complexion, sad brown hair, as you may find more at large in this book.

Signs of recovery, was first *Saturn* Lord of the ascendant, being his significator is strong as being in his own house, and is more strong than *Mars* who is the afflicting Planet. Secondly the *Moon* separates from *Mars*, and applies first to *Venus*, and from thence to the *Sun* and *Jupiter*, all fortunes. Thirdly, the *Moon* is increasing in light. Fourthly neither the *Moon*, or *Saturn* are combust ; Planets are said to be combust, when they are not elongated eight *deg*. thirty *min*. from the *Sun*. Fifthly, she is not in that part of the Zodiac called *via combusta*, which is from the middle of *Libra* to the middle of *Scorpio*. Lastly, *Venus*

Lady of the fourth house, which usually shows the end of all things of this nature, was in friendly aspect to the Moon, at the time of decumbiture ; all of which are arguments of recovery. The time when follows, First, the angles of the figure are part fixed, and part common. Secondly, the Moon was in a common sign which argues, that the grief was not perfectly acute, nor yet chronic, but between both and so it proved, for upon the last critical day the fever left him, at which time the Moon came to the place, she was in at the decumbiture *viz.* to the ninth *deg.* of *Sagittarius* : yet notwithstanding at the last critical time he had a very strong fit the Moon being then in square to Mars ; but *Venus* fortune and Lady of the fourth house, being in friendly aspect to the Moon, and she together with *Saturn* being both more strong than Mars, who was the afflicting Planet, put an end to this sickness at the time aforesaid.

The next thing to consider, is to discover the grief, and from what cause ; and likewise what infirmities he was naturally subject to from the birth : Now concerning the present acute grief, I found the Moon being in the sign *Sagitary*, was the platic square of Mars afflicted, for between the sign *Virgo*, the place where Mars is, and the sign *Sagitary*, the place where the Moon is, contains ninety *deg.* which number makes a square had the Moon been but one degree in the sign *Sagitary* yet that would have been a platic square, for if we consider the moiety of each Orb, there will be ten *deg.* allotted, at which time and distance, the influence of those Planets operate, both before and after any aspect. Now to know what the present distemper was by reason it was an acute grief ; you must find out the place in this book entitled, the Moon in *Sagittary*, of Mars oppressed, which argues a high and strong fever with the flux or lask and choleric passions ; the pulses few and faint beating slowly, his blood over heated. The bright star of the Harp [Wega] and the Star called the Swans-bill [Albireo], both of the nature of Mars and *Jupiter* in the ascendant made the fever the more violent : The cause of this sickness was from inordinate exercise ; surfeiting, or too much repletion, as you may find more at large at the place aforesaid.

[The way of recovery was by application Antipathetical to *Mars* the afflicting planet by reason that *Venus* was more strong in essential dignities, as being in her house. Now in regard that *Mars* is by nature hot and dry, I made choice of such herbs and other remedies, which were cold and moist ; wherefore I advised that such decoctions, syrups, or cordials, which were administered should be cooling and cleansing, also glisters the like, ever remembering as in this, so in all other cures, to fortify the heart and vital spirits with herbs under the dominion of the *Sun* : Would the Patient have been persuaded to let blood, the fever would without question have left him, upon the second critical time, the *Moon* meeting then with the friendly aspect of *Venus* a fortune and strong.

Note, That as we give judgements by the *Sun* and *Moon* afflicted, in acute and chronic griefs so by the same rules you may give judgement by the Lord of the ascendant or sixth house afflicted.

Example, In the last figure, *Mercury* being Lord of the sixth house, and in the sign *Libra*, is in platic square to *Saturn*, and conjunction of the *Sun*, who is much of the nature of *Mars*, only the *Sun* strikes more upon the vital spirits : Now according to the rule in giving judgement by the *Moon* afflicted in the sign *Libra*, it shows a feverish distemper and blood over heated, occasioned from surfeiting.

The next thing to consider is to know, what infirmities naturally he was subject to from the birth. In this question judgement must be given from the ascendant, sixth house, and their Lords afflicted ; first the ascendant is in no way afflicted, save only by the presence of *Saturn*, who is Lord thereof : Now in this question *Saturn* is not accounted an enemy, notwithstanding he is naturally evil, as being in his own house, and Lord of the sick man's person, for according to the old saying, the devil will not hurt his own. Also the sixth house is no way afflicted, wherefore we have only *Mercury* Lord of the sixth to consider herein, and he I find is in *Libra* in platic conjunction of *Venus* Lady of the fourth. Now any planet although he be naturally a fortune may afflict so well, as the infortunes being Lord or Lady of the fourth, sixth, eighth, or twelfth houses, for every planet must do his Office ; to know what the grief is you must take notice of the sign, where *Mercury* Lord of the sixth house is, *viz.* in *Libra*, and what parts of the body is signified thereby, also what griefs or infirmities are under the dominion of *Venus* : First under the sign *Libra* is reins and loins, and under *Venus* is also the reins together with back, belly and members of generation and passages of urine. To my knowledge he has for many years past been ofttimes perplexed with difficulty of making water, and with pains in his reins, back, and belly. What I have written I presume will be sufficient to instruct the learner, but practice and experience will be the only means to enlarge the practitioner's judgement herein, for 'tis impossible for any man to write, be he never so curious and exact in any art, but that somewhat may be added to it.

Observations concerning the Ascendant

That which I have found by daily practice and experience, is carefully to erect your figure (either for the time of decumbiture, or the time of any strong fit, or when the Patient was more than ordinarily sick or afflicted, or for the time when the urine is brought, or when you go to visit the patient) that the Ascendant together with its Lord may exactly personate the Sick, for if neither the ascendant nor the Lord thereof agrees in shape, complexion, and hair with the body of the Sick, you

Observations Concerning the Ascendant 51

cannot safely give judgement by a figure of twelve houses, especially in many infirmities, as I have often experienced ; for the first, fourth, sixth, eighth, and twelfth houses will be especially concerned therein ; wherefore if you fail in the first foundation, the whole building must needs be obstructed and out of order.

Example, In the decumbiture figure before mentioned, had I erected the figure but for one hour sooner, *Sagitary* would have ascended, whereof *Jupiter* is Lord, and then the person of the sick must have been described accordingly. Now *Jupiter* signifies a man of an upright and tall stature, complexion ruddy, face oval, full, and fleshy, and a kind of a brune brown hair : Also the sign *Sagitary* represents a man much after the same shape and likeness, by which it appears what a vast difference it might produce by taking a wrong ascendant, both in regard of the personal shape, and likewise in the discovery of the grief of the sick : Whereas it appears by taking the true ascendant, that it does not only delineate his person, as is before expressed, but does] exactly discover his present distemper, and natural infirmities : For let the time of decumbiture or the time for receipt of the urine, or the time of any strong fit be brought, and the Artist never so curious by enquiry, except by chance, he shall not get the true ascendant, for many reasons may be objected to the contrary : First clocks may fail, and so sick persons will hold out longer than others before complaint, and the urine may by the messenger be hastened, or retarded, you see one hour makes a mighty alteration. I shall quote another *Example,* Suppose a Man or Woman, who is under the dominion of *Sol* Lord of *Leo*, should fall sick, which represents one of a large stature, fat, full, and fleshy, complexion sanguine, and yellowish hair. Now perhaps when the urine is brought, or through mistakes of clocks or time, *Gemini* should ascend, whereof *Mercury* is Lord, what a mighty difference could this produce : For the planet *Mercury* represents one of an upright and tall stature, spare body, long face and nose, of a dark swarthy complexion, and sad hair : Also the sign *Gemini* signifies a tall body, a dark and obscure complexion, and sad or black hair. I could instance many more, wherefore advise all practitioners in this art so to vary their ascendant, that it together with its Lord or planet posited in the ascendant may exactly personate the Sick, without which no true judgment can be given especially in many chronic griefs or infirmities, and in case of Witchcraft and Sorcery.

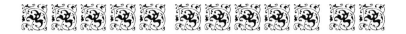

Some brief Rules concerning long and short sicknesses ; and whether the Patient is like to live or die.

First of long or short Sickness

1 A fixed sign on the Cusp of the sixth, or the Lord of the sixth, or Lord of the Ascendant, or the *Moon* in acute ; or *Sun* in Chronic griefs be in fixed signs afflicted by the malevolent Planets, or by the Lord of the 12, 8, or 4th, argues long and lasting griefs or infirmities ; if adhering to a partile aspect, the grief increases ; if drawing from partile aspect, the grief diminishes : Also fixed signs gives months, and sometimes years before recovery ; common signs gives weeks, and sometimes months, moveable days or weeks before recovery. Now concerning the number of days, weeks, months or years, you must observe how many degrees is wanting before the influence is over, accounting by the moiety of their Orbs, and so many months, weeks, days or years it will be before recovery ; but if the figure shows death, then you must account how many degrees is wanting to make the partile aspect of the principal Significators, and so account so many days, weeks, months or years before the time of death.

   2 The principal Significator of the Sick changing his sign, argues a change of the disease, either for life or death.

3 The latter degrees of a sign on the Cusp of the sixth House, or the Significator of the Sick in the latter degrees of a sign argues a sudden change either for life or death.

4 The Lord of the Ascendant, or principal significator of the sick person, being stronger then the afflicting planets shows recovery, in moveable signs the sooner ; but if the afflicting Planets be strong, and the principal Significator of the Sick weak, more especially if the afflicting Planets has relation to the eighth or fourth Houses, it shows death.

5 If the Lord of the Ascendant, or Lord of the sixth, or if the ☽ in acute, or *Sun* in Chronic griefs be afflicted in Azimene degrees, it shows a continued sickness, if not sudden death.

6 If the Lord of the Ascendant, or principal Significator of the sick turn retrograde, it shows a relapse, and the cure goes backward.

7 The Lord of the Ascendant, or principal Significator of the sick strong, swift in motion, with a fortune attending, especially in a moveable sign, shows a speedy recovery.

Lastly, We must heed the nature of the disease, for strong Fevers, Convulsions, Apoplexies, risings in the Throat, with some pestilential infirmities, and such like desperate griefs, will sooner terminate, than such which are usually lasting, as Consumptions, Dropsies, Agues, Gouts, and such like.

Some brief Rules concerning recovery.

First, A fortune, or the ☽ in acute, or ☉ in Chronic griefs strong in the Ascendant, and not afflicted, nor yet being Lord of the sixth, eighth or twelfth Houses, shows recovery.

Secondly, The Lord of the Ascendant strong, and more strong than the afflicting Planets, shows recovery.

Thirdly, The Lord of the Ascendant, or the ☽ in acute, or ☉ in Chronic griefs joined to, or friendly aspect with a fortune, or applying to a fortune, shows recovery.

Fourthly, The ☽ increasing in light, swift in motion, and strong applying to a fortune in acute griefs, shows recovery.

Fifthly, If the Lord of the ascendant dispossess of the afflicting Planet, especially being equal in strength, shows recovery.

Signs of Death.

First, The Lord of the Ascendant weak and afflicted by the malevolent Planets, and no fortune interposing, shows death.

Secondly, The Lord of the ascendant, or the ☽ afflicted in the fourth or eighth, or by the Lord of the eighth, argues death, or if the Lord of the eighth be in the ascendant.

Thirdly, The Lord of the ascendant combust in the ascendant, fourth, sixth, eighth, or twelfth, or in the way called *Via Combusta*, shows death.

Fourthly, If the ☽ in acute, or ☉ in Chronic griefs is afflicted by the infortunes, or by the Lord of the eighth or fourth, no fortune interposing their friendly rays, more especially if the Lord of the ascendant be weak ; it shows death.

Fifthly, The ascendant, or Lord of the ascendant, or the ☽ in acute, or the ☉ in Chronic griefs meeting with fixed stars of the nature of the infortunes, no fortune interposing his friendly rays, shows death.

Sixthly, The ☽ applying to combustion in the ascendant, fourth, sixth, eighth, or twelfth houses, or *Via combusta*, shows death.

Seventhly, The ☽ applying from the Lord of the ascendant to the Lord of the eighth, and the Lord of the ascendant weak, shows death.

Eighthly, An eclipse of the ☽ in acute, or of the Sun in Chronic griefs upon a critical day, and the Lord of the ascendant weak, no fortune strong interposing their friendly rays, shows death, generally in all decumbitures, the nearer the afflicting Planets are to the earth, the worst.

The bodily shape and infirmities attributed to the Twelve Signs.

Aries ♈ signifies one of a reasonable stature, dry body, strong limbs, and big bones, but not fat, somewhat long face and neck, complexion somewhat brown, their hair and eyebrows inclining to blackness : the diseases incident to this Sign is Pushes, Whelks, Polypus, or Noli me tangere. All diseases which proceed from the head, as Convulsions, dead Palsies, Cramps, Madness, Vertigo, Migraines, Falling Sickness, and such like.

Taurus ♉ signifies one short, but full and well set, full face and eyes, broad forehead, large strong shoulders, full hands, thick lips, and black rugged hair ; under this Sign are all diseases incident to the throat, as Kings Evil, Quinzies, Fluxes of Rheums falling from the head into the throat, Impostumes and Wens in the neck.

Gemini ♊ those persons usually who are under the dominion of this Sign, are tall and straight of body, with long arms, of a dark sanguine complexion, and blackish hair, their body strong and active ; under this Sign are all diseases in the arms, hands and shoulders, with windiness in the veins, corrupted blood, sometimes it produces distempered fancies.

Cancer ♋ signifies one of a low and small stature, bigger made from the middle upwards than downwards, face big and round, of a whitish pale complexion, sad brown hair, one apt to be sickly ; under this Sign are all imperfections of the breast and stomach, as Cancers, Ptisick, Salt flegm, rotten Coughs, weak digestion, cold stomach, dropsical humors, and Impostumations.

Leo ♌ signifies one of a large fair stature, full and fleshy, narrow sides, and broad shoulders, full and great eyes, sometimes goggle-eyed, yellow or dark flaxen hair, sometimes curling, of a sanguine or ruddy complexion ; under this Sign are all tremblings or passions of the heart, violent burning Fevers, pains either at the heart or back, sore eyes, Plague, Pestilence, and Yellow Jaundies.

Virgo ♍ signifies one of a mean stature, but well composed, a brown ruddy complexion, black hair, shrill and small voice, well favoured, but not very beautiful : The diseases which are incident to this sign, are all such which belong to the belly, as obstructions in the bowels, and miseraicks, worms, wind, Colic, Spleen, Hypochondriac Melancholy, and such like.

Libra ♎ personates one of a well framed body, straight and tall, a round and beautiful visage, a pure sanguine complexion but not very high coloured, the hair yellowish or sandy-brown, and somewhat smooth ; under this Sign are all diseases of the reins and kidneys, also all diseases proceeding from wind, and corruption of blood.

Scorpio ♏ signifies one of a middle stature, strong, full, and well set, somewhat broad-faced, of a muddy or darkish complexion, sad or black hair, bow-legged, short-necked, and somewhat hairy : The diseases incident to this Sign, are Ulcers, Inflammations, Gravel or Stone in the Bladder, all imperfections and difficulties of Urine, Ruptures, Hemorrhoids, the French Pox, and Running of the Reins, Priapism, and all diseases which infect the Privies both of men and women.

Sagitary ♐ signifies one of a fair stature, and strong body, long face, but full and fleshy, complexion sanguine or ruddy, the hair a kind of Chestnut colour ; the diseases which are under this Sign are fevers, and such infirmities which are occasioned through heat of blood : The Sciatica, and all pains in the Hips and Thighs, falls from horses, and hurts by four-footed beasts.

Capricorn ♑ signifies one rather short than tall, narrow, long face, thin beard, black hair, narrow breast, small neck, complexion swarthy ; under this Sign are all diseases in the Knees and Hams, Leprosies, Itch and Scabs, all diseases of melancholy, all scurrilous tumors, sprains, fractures and dislocations.

Aquary ♒ represents one of a thick square corporature, strong and well composed, not very tall, visage long, complexion fair and clear, hair sandy-coloured, but if ♄ be in this House at the birth, then black hair, and the complexion will be more sanguine, with distorted teeth ; under this Sign are all diseases incident to the legs and ankles, and all melancholy winds coagulated in the veins and blood ; also Cramps.

Pisces ♓ represents one of a short stature, not decent, but rather ill composed, a large face, complexion pale, the body fleshy or swelling, and somewhat incurvating with the head ; the diseases subject to this sign are all lameness, and aches incident to the feet, and all diseases coming of salt phlegm, and mixed humors, all blood putrefied, as Scabs, Itch and Botches, or breakings out about the body, Small Pox and Measles ; also all cold and moist diseases, and such which come of catching cold and wet at the feet.

The bodily shape, with the parts and members of the body and diseases which the Planets generally rule

♄ *Saturn* represents one of a middle stature, broad and large shoulders, sometimes crooked, his thighs lean, his feet and knees indecent, many times hitting or shovelling one against the other, broad forehead, eyes little, complexion muddy or swarthy, looking downward, thick lips and nose, thin beard, black hair : Diseases and sicknesses subject to this Planet are Quartan Agues, and diseases proceeding from cold, dry, and melancholy distempers ; the retentive faculties, all impediments in the right ear, and teeth, also Rheums, Consumptions, Black Jaundies, Palsies, tremblings, and vain fears, Dropsies, the hand and feet Gout, the Spleen and bones.

♃ *Jupiter* signifies one of an upright and tall stature, a large deep belly, thighs and legs strong proportioned, his feet long, face oval, full and fleshy, complexion brown, ruddy, and lovely high forehead, his hair soft, and a kind of a brown, much beard, his speech sober : The diseases under this Planet are Pleurisies, and all infirmities in the liver, lungs, ribs, sides, veins, blood ; the digestive faculty, Cramps, pain in the back-bone, Squinzies, windiness, and putrefaction in the blood, Fevers proceeding from wind, and ill blood.

♂ *Mars* signifies one of a middle stature, body strong, big bones, not fat visage, round complexion, ruddy, the hair between red and sandy brown, crisping or curling, hazel eyes, a bold confident man or woman, and fearless : The sicknesses incident to this Planet are tertain Fevers, and pestilent burning Fevers, the Plague, Bloody Flux, Small Pox, all diseases of choler, the Shingles, Gall, and left ear phrensies, and sudden distempers in the head, Carbuncles, Fistulas, all fears and hurts by iron.

☉ *Sun* Those who are under the Sun are of a strong large corporature, and well composed body, fat and fleshy, of a yellow saffron ruddy complexion, goggle or large eyes, hair yellowish : The sicknesses under this Planet are all diseases of the heart and brain, palpitations, tremblings, sudden swoundings, Catarrhs, the Nerves and Arteries, the right eye of men, the left eye of women, and vital spirit of both ; all infirmities of the eyes, and diseases of the mouth, rotten Fevers, and stinking breaths.

♀ *Venus* signifies one somewhat short, but full and well set, fat and fleshy face, round complexion, dark, but lovely light brown hair, and smooth, a rowling eye, and full of amorous enticements, a body well shaped, and delightful : Sicknesses under this Planet, are all diseases of the Matrix, and members of Generation, Running of the Reins, French Pox, also griefs of the Belly, Back, and Navel, any disease arising by inordinate lust, Priapism, Diabetes, or pissing disease, Hernias, and impotency in the act of Generation, the throat, women's breasts, and the milk in them.

☿ *Mercury* denotes one tall of stature, spare body, long arms and hands, long face and nose, thin lips, little hair on his chin, but pretty store on his head, inclining to blackness, an olive or sallow complexion, eyes between black and grey, oft times much partaking of the Planet he is joined withal : Sicknesses under this Planet, are all diseases of the brain, as Madness, Vertigoes, Lethargies, or giddiness in the head, Ptisick, stammering, memory, dry coughs, snuffling in the head or nose, dumbness, all evils in the fancy, or intellectual parts, and tongue, the Nerves, the defects of the Uvula, or Gargareon.

☽ *Moon* The Moon generally represents one of a fair stature, phlegmatic, full, fat, and fleshy round face, complexion white, lowring looks, hair light brown, grey eyes : Sicknesses and diseases are Apoplexies, Palsy, Colic, Bellyache, the Menstrues in women, Dropsies, Fluxes of the Belly, all cold Rheumatic diseases, and cold Stomach, Surfeits, rotten Coughs, Convulsions, Falling-Sickness, Kings Evil, Apostems, Small Pox and Measles, the Colic, Bladder, and Members of Generation.

Concerning what effects the Moon works in any of the twelve Signs upon the Body of the Sick, she being afflicted by the Conjunction, Square, or opposition Aspects of Mars at the decumbiture.

Note, *that the Sun afflicting the Moon, works near the same effects, only the* ☉ *strikes more upon the Heart and Vital Spirits.*

The ☽ Moon *in* ♈ Aries *of* ♂ Mars *afflicted or oppressed.*

If at the time of Decumbiture the Moon be in ♈ *Aries* of ♂ or ☉ oppressed either by ♂ □ or ☍, then the Sick shall be tormented with continual Fevers, with little or no rest or quietness, a continued extreme thirst, and dryness of the tongue and breast, an inflammation of the Liver, tending to a Phrensie, high and inordinate Pulses, sometimes a deprivation of senses, and the Patient ready to run mad, or has some extreme pain or grief in their belly, or small guts, occasioned by choleric obstructions : The original cause of this disease shall proceed from a distempered affection of the Membranes, or pellets of the brain, and excess of choleric matter. If *Venus* be stronger then *Mars*, then cooling remedies will be suitable ; however 'twill be necessary to let blood. Concerning the way how to cure each distemper, is set down elsewhere in this book.

The Moon *in* Taurus *of Mars afflicted.*

Those that take their bed under such configuration, as aforesaid, shall be afflicted with a continued Fever, the whole frame of the body obstructed, with an inflammation of the

Throat, Neck, and hinder part thereof, and ache of the bones ; also insomnia, or inordinate watching, very thirsty, longing after cooling things : Oft time the sick will be afflicted with the Strangury, or Stone, with Gravel in the Reins and Kidneys, pestilent sore throats, or hoarseness, or some ill matter settled there : The cause is from much ill blood, choler, and sweet flegm.

The Moon in Gemini of Mars oppressed.

Those who take their bed under this configuration, shall be afflicted with a violent burning Fever, and with obstructions, their blood extreme windy and corrupted, some great pains or lameness in their arms or Joints, the pulses long and inordinate ; oft-times the Patient is troubled with the Stone or heat in the Reins, and sometimes spitting of blood : The cause of this distemper usually is from ingurgitation, or too much drinking of strong Wine or Beer, and some choleric matter.

The Moon in Cancer of Mars oppressed.

Those that take their bed when the ☽ is in *Cancer* of *Mars* afflicted, the sick will be troubled with much phlegm, and ill matter settled at their Breast and Stomach ; also with eversion, and turning of the Ventricle, oft-times desiring to vomit, with some defect in the blood : This disease comes from surfeiting, or too much ingurgitation, and oft-times turns to a looseness, or a rotten Cough, and sometimes spitting blood.

The Moon in Leo of Mars oppressed.

Those who take their bed when the Moon is in *Leo* of *Mars* afflicted, shall be subject to a strong Fever, with a disturbed brain, and strong raging fits ; also they will be subject to much drowsiness and heaviness all over their body ; also the heart oppressed with faintness and swounding fits, and the party almost raging mad, with little or no appetite : The cause of this distemper is from excess of choler, and blood abounding, over-heated.

The Moon in Virgo of Mars oppressed.

Those who take their bed under this configuration, shall be subject to a Flux in the belly, small Fevers, the Pulse remiss, aversion of the Ventricle, also tormented with wind in the Belly or Guts, and Cholic, bad stomach many times, weakness or pains in the legs near the ankles ; the cause from original choler, melancholy, and sharp fretting humors.

The Moon in Libra of Mars oppressed.

Those who take their bed, the Moon being in ♎ of ♂ oppressed, will be subject to an inflammation all over the body, also Feverish, unapt to sleep, their Pulses high, troubled with wind and plenitude of blood, many times they have the stone or gravel in the kidneys or great heat therein : The cause is from surfeiting or disorder in diet, also plenitude of blood.

The Moon in Scorpio of Mars oppressed.

Those who take their bed, the *Moon* being in *Scorpio* of *Mars* oppressed, argues that the sick is afflicted, or has some grievous infirmity in their privy parts. If children or Young-people, then it argues the small-pox or measles. Also it shows (more especially in times of pestilential diseases) the pestilence, or some poisonous or pestilential grief : many times it causes boils or scabiness to break forth. The cause is from blood extremely corrupted, or from some infectious and poisonous grief, accidentally taken into the body by smell or taste.

The Moon in Sagitary of Mars oppressed.

Those, who take their bed the Moon being in *Sagitary* of *Mars* oppressed shall be tormented with high fevers, and choleric passions, with the flux or lask, the pulses few and faint, the sick burns extremely many times, it shows the hand and foot gout with breaking out, and sore throats, sometimes sharp rheums offend their eyes. The cause is from surfeiting or gluttony, or too much repletion. Also from inordinate exercise, and blood over-heated.

The Moon in Capricorn of Mars oppressed.

Those who take their bed, the Moon being in *Capricorn* of *Mars* oppressed, shall be troubled with excess of choler, and with great desire to vomit, no perfect concoction, and oft returning fevers, a puffing up the sinews, and a flux of the belly immediately follows an inflammation of the breast ; some exulceration in a Choleric humour offends the party in his hands or joints of his fingers, also the sick is inclining to the yellow jaundies. Their blood all over the body disaffected. The cause is from choler, and evil digestion, and blood corrupted.

The Moon in Aquary of Mars oppressed.

Those who take their bed the Moon being in *Aquary* of *Mars* oppressed, are troubled with swooning fits, and pained at the heart, and are very feverish, pulses are high, and the blood swelling in all their veins, oft-times complaining of great pain in their breast, drawing their wind with great difficulty. The cause is from most sharp and violent affections or vehement passions.

The Moon in Pisces of Mars oppressed.

Those who take their bed when the *Moon* is in *Pisces* of *Mars* afflicted shall be tormented with sharp burning fevers and vehement thirst, and usually oppressed with a violent looseness, complaining of great pain in their bellies, or an extraordinary rotten cough, also a deflux of rheum falling from the head to the throat, they being near suffocated therewith, their bellies swollen and in danger of a dropsy, oft-times they are troubled with itching and a salt humor in the blood. The cause of the distemper is from too much ingurgitation, and drinking of wine and strong drinks, and the body abounding with choler, and salt phlegm, and blood corrupted occasioned by disorder.

Concerning what effects the Moon works in any of the twelve Signs, upon the body of the Sick, She being afflicted by the Conjunction, Square or Opposition of Saturn at the time of decumbiture.

Note, That Mercury afflicting the Moon works the same effects only he strikes somewhat more upon the brain and nerves.

The Moon in Aries of Saturn or Mercury oppressed.

THose who take their bed, the *Moon* being in *Aries* of *Saturn* or *Mercury* oppressed, shall be troubled with headache, and a distillation of Rheums falling from the head into the throat and wind pipe, also a stuffing in the head, with dullness of the eyes, inordinate drowsiness, and dullness of mind, and bad stomach, intemperate sweats, being hot within and cold without, more afflicted in the night than by day. The occasion of this distemper is from great cold taken, and want of exercise, and sometimes by eating trash contrary to Nature.

The Moon in Taurus *of* Saturn *or* Mercury *oppressed.*

Those who take their bed, the *Moon* being in *Taurus* of *Saturn* or *Mercury* oppressed, shall be feverish proceeding from obstructions and distempers of the precordiacs and arteries, *viz.* of the inward parts near the heart, liver, and lungs, some ulceration there abouts, their pulses are lofty and high, and an inflammation of the whole body. The disease proceeds from too much luxury, or from surfeiting or inordinate repletion, also melancholy and ill diet.

The Moon in Gemini *of* Saturn *or* Mercury *oppressed,*

Those who take their bed under this configuration shall be in danger of a fever, and the pain disperses itself all over the body, but principally in the Arteries and joints : Also the Sick inclines to a Consumption : the vitals much afflicted, the pulse low and little : also they will be subject to frequent sweatings with Symptoms of the Spleen. The disease more troublesome in the night than in the day. The cause of this distemper is from much waiting, weariness of the mind, and overburdening with multiplicity of affairs, excess of labour, or violent exercise.

The Moon in Cancer *of* Saturn *or* Mercury *oppressed.*

Those who take their bed, the *Moon* being in *Cancer* of *Saturn* oppressed, shall be afflicted in the breast with tough melancholy matter or thick flegm : also troubled with Coughs, Catharrs, hoarseness, and a distillation of Rheums or Humours falling into the breast, their pipes are narrow and obstructed, inordinate fevers, pulses little and low, oft-times a Quotidian, but now especially a Quartan Ague follows with bellyache, or some infirmities in the reins or Secrets. If the *Moon* be decreasing and near the body of *Saturn*, the sickness is like to be long and lasting. The cause is from great cold and inordinate eating or drinking, and want of moderate exercise.

The Moon *in* Leo *of* Saturn *or* Mercury *oppressed.*

Those who take their bed, the *Moon* being in *Leo* of *Saturn* oppressed, shall be oppressed with much heat in the breast and intension of the heart strings, with augmenting fevers, the pulses keeping no course, annoyed with external and internal heat : also great faintness of heart or swooning fits, after some time, if not cured the sick will be subject to the black jaundies. The cause is from grief taken, and ill melancholy blood.

The Moon *in* Virgo *of* Saturn *or* Mercury *oppressed.*

Those who take their beds, when the *Moon* is in *Virgo* of *Saturn* oppressed, shall be troubled with in ordinate fevers, pricking or shooting under the ribs : also vicious phlegm obstructing the bowels, sometimes the wind cholic afflicts them : also the gout and aches in the thighs and feet : I oft-times find they are much troubled with worms. The cause of this distemper is usually from crudities, and evil digestion in the stomach and contrary diet.

The Moon *in* Libra *of* Saturn *or* Mercury *oppressed.*

Those who take their bed, when the *Moon* is in *Libra* of *Saturn* or *Mercury* oppressed shall be troubled with pains of the head, breast, and stomach disaffected ; the cough, hoarseness and distillation of rheums shall afflict them, and loss of Appetite, small fevers troubling them by night, oft-times great pains in their joints, knees, and thighs : also some defect in their reins, kidneys, and bladder. The cause is originally from surfeiting or gluttony and meat not fully digested or excess of Venery.

The Moon in Scorpio of Saturn or Mercury oppressed.

Those who take their bed, the *Moon* being in *Scorpio* of *Saturn* afflicted, shall be subject to some defects in their secret parts, hemorrhoids, piles, or some exulceration, their no retention of urine, oft-times vexed with the stone or stop in the bladder, sometimes if a man the gonorrhea, if a woman too much of menstrues. The cause is of corrupt phlegm, or disorder of body.

The Moon in Sagitary of Saturn or Mercury oppressed.

Those who take their bed, when the *Moon* is in *Sagittary* of *Saturn* oppressed, shall be tormented with defluction of thin sharp humors, and aches of the sinews, and arteries, extremities of heat and cold, and oft-times a double access of a fever, and most commonly a violent burning fever at the first being ill. The cause is from blood infected with choler and melancholy, and sometimes by great painstaking or violent exercise and cold taken thereupon.

The Moon in Capricorn of Saturn or Mercury oppressed.

Those who take their bed, with the *Moon* is in *Capricorn* of *Saturn* oppressed shall be afflicted with heaviness at the breast and stomach, and difficulty of breathing, and dry Coughs, their lungs oppressed, more pained by night than day, with intended fevers, oft times troubled with headache, and noise in their head. The cause is from great cold, melancholy and disorderly diet.

The Moon in Aquary of Saturn or Mercury oppressed.

Those who take their bed the Moon being in the sign Aquary of Saturn or Mercury, afflicted, shall be troubled with much melancholy, winds coagulated in the veins, the malady ceases on them unequally with remission and intension, their heads pained with wind or noise. Also troubled with faint fits or passion of the heart, sometimes a sore throat, or troubled with a rising there, being in danger of suffocation. The cause is from excess of labour, want of sleep whereby to refresh nature, and much trouble of mind.

The Moon in Pisces of Saturn or Mercury oppressed.

Those who take their bed, when the Moon is in Pisces, of Saturn oppressed shall be troubled with much sighing and pricking or shooting of the breast and under the paps, and continual augmenting fevers, with extentions of the precordiacs and heart-strings, or arteries ; also their throat is oppressed with thick phlegm, and their breast with a rotten cough, and store of watery matter lodging there. The cause is from extremity of cold taken by bathing, or otherwise by much wet.

The Way to make diet drinks by decoctions or to extract the Spirits of Plants or Herbs : Also to make Syrups, Lohochs, or Lambatives, Pills, Glisters, Fumes, Suffumigations, Cataplasms, Ointments, Baths : Also the making and administrating of Purgations and vomits, and concerning blood-letting, &c.

Concerning Decoctions and Diet-drinks.

Having by the Rules elsewhere expressed in this Book collected the herbs together suitable to the cure according to their virtues and numbers, always remembering in all cures to fortify the heart with herbs proper, you must take the herbs and chop them small : But to all diet drinks I usually add as follows, to make it the more strong and useful, *viz.* raisins, currants, (sometimes figs), liquorice, and aniseed, and if the Patient be much troubled with wind, then you may also put into it sweet fennel-seed, coriander-seed and such like, which are good to expel wind. These additions must be bruised well in a mortar, and so boiled with the herbs, when it's boiling you must keep them close covered, whereby to keep in the spirit, you may boil these herbs, with the addition in beer or ale. If you desire to make it strong and nutritive, then when it is new boiled you may put into it white wine, muscatel, or brandy, according to the temper of the Patient. A good handful of all sorts of herbs put together will be sufficient for three or four gallons of liquor ; you may let it boil until a fourth part or thereabouts be wasted, for if you keep it close covered it will not waste very much in the boiling : Now of this diet drink we usually give the Patient thereof three times a day, *viz.* morning, afternoon and at night, and every morning about an hour after they have taken the diet drink, you must give the Patient water gruel or broth made with either the same herbs, or other herbs which are suitable to the Cure, according to their virtues and numbers.

How to extract the Spirits of Plants and Herbs.

If the Patient be weak, and must take small quantities, then you must do as follows, having collected the herbs together suitable to the cure, shred them small with the addition according as in the decoction aforesaid, and put them into a limbeck still ; and put into it a quantity of beer or ale with some white wine, muscatel, and brandy to make it proportionable to the quantity of liquor and herbs before expressed, *viz.* a good handful of herbs with the additions to two quarts or better of liquor, this will keep a long time. There is yet another way to extract the Spirit as follows. Take the herbs with the additions, being shred small and bruised, put them into warm water, and put some berm in it, let it work three days, as does beer, and then distill it in a limbeck still, if you desire to have it strong you may put brandy or Spirit of Wine in it, and put fresh herbs to it, and still it over again.

The way to make Syrups.

Take the Roses, herbs or flowers, and bruise them, put them into a convenient quantity of fair water, my usual dose is about three pints of water to a pound of flowers, roses, or herbs : let the water be hot, and let it stand with the herbs or flowers in it, about twelve hours, then strain it and infuse more of the same herbs or flowers, and heat more water and put to it ; you must sometimes infuse the roses, herbs, or flowers whole without bruising to make it have the smell of the plant : The more of the roses, herbs, or flowers you infuse into the liquor, the stronger it will be, and the oftener you infuse the better : The

Concerning Lohochs or Lambatives   73

last infusions I usually boil, and then gently strain it, and to every pint of liquor add a pound of the best Sugar at the least, you must simmer it over the fire, until it be a Syrup, you may know when 'tis enough by cooling some in a spoon, when 'tis made you must keep it in glasses or stone pots, bound over only with paper, or such like, you must not stop it close with cork, lest it break the glass.

Concerning Lohochs or Lambatives the making and use.

Having made your election of such herbs, which are of virtue to cure, such inward defects required, shred and boil them by way of decoction, and when you have strained it, put twice its weight of honey or sugar, and so boil it to a Lohoch, which is somewhat thicker than a Syrup, if the grief be of phlegm, then honey is best. These lambatives are usually taken with a liquorice stick. And are most usually taken for inflammations and ulcers in the lungs, Coughs, Asthmas and difficulty of breath, and such like infirmities.

Concerning Pills their making and use.

All kinds of Pills are made only by beating the substantial matter into a powder, and so with syrup (or little gum *Tragacanth* dissolved in distilled water) made up into Pills. They are usually taken at night. If it be only to cause the Patient to go to stool the next day, then so much aloe as will heap on a two pence for a strong body or less for a weak body mixed with a little myrrh and saffron will be enough, these Pills are also good for the head and stomach. There are many sorts of Pills made for several infirmities, as you may find in the *London Dispensary*, to which I shall refer you. I confess I seldom use any Pills, except what I have mentioned ; for I find the Astrological way of cure by herbs does (if rightly applied) cure all distempers, and griefs whatsoever, loosen the body and allay any pain of the head, and the like as you shall find in this book, yet sometimes when the patient is bound in body and the distemper requires a decoction made of such herbs, which are commonly heating, and so for the most part binding, such as are palpitations, convulsions, palsies, apoplexies, and such like. Then I usually give the Patient Pills at night made as aforesaid, if need require.

Concerning Glisters

If the Patient be much afflicted in the belly and Guts, or is very costive in body, as sometimes it will fall out, more especially when the grief requires herbs heating and binding to work their cure, then I usually apply Glisters and ointments made of such herbs, which are antipathetical to the afflicting Planet : But most especially such herbs, which are good to comfort the heart, to expel poison, and cleanse the Guts. Also you must be careful that the herbs be gathered at the right planetary hours, not omitting their numbers which belong to each Planet. When you have gotten the herbs together, shred them small, and boil them in milk, together with such seeds and roots, which are good to expel winds, about a pint and a half of milk boiled until it be near half wasted will be enough, for any reasonable man or woman : after its boiled and strained I usually put into it three or four spoonfuls of sallet oil, and a spoonful of honey or coarse sugar. And so give it the Patient blood warm. But my usual way is first to give the Patient a suppository made of *Sal-Gem* to bring them first to stool, by which means I find the Glister works the more effectively upon the humour offending. For many times if no suppository be first given the glisters will not stay, by reason the Patient cannot keep them in their body.

Concerning Fumes.

If the head and brain be disaffected by reason of superfluous moisture then fumes are proper to used by reason they have a drying quality, provided they be made antipathetical to the afflicting planet ; you must shred, bruise, and dry those herbs, plants, or roots, which you intend to use, and to bring them into powder ; and when you intend to fume their heads put some of this powder upon hot coals and let the Patients hold their heads over it, twice a day is enough, *viz.* morning and evening. They must be careful to keep their head and feet warm.

Concerning Suffumigations

If the head and brain be disaffected by reason of great draught, be it hot or cold draught, you must make choice of such herbs according to their virtues and numbers, which are antipathetical to the afflicting Planet, shred them small and boil them, either in strong beer, ale, or strong malted water, and while it is hot, let the Patients hold their head over it, and be careful they take no cold afterwards.

Concerning Cataplasms

Cataplasms are oft-times used to help cure Agues and sometimes to apply to the feet to draw from the head, and more especially in such infirmities and defects wherein the Nerves and arteries are concerned being laid to the pulse, neck, and other parts of the body, as occasion is offered. I commonly use them in convulsions, apoplexies, palpitations, and such like distempers. The way to make them is thus, you must make choice of such herbs according to their virtues and numbers, which are good to cure the grief as you shall find in this book, shred them small and pound them in a mortar, with a quantity of white Salt, and a few raisins, honey, a little Venus turpentine, or burgundy pitch to make it hold together, you must lay it on hot.

Concerning Ointments.

Those Ointments which are made heating must be made with sallet-Oil, and those Ointments, which are cooling must be made with either neats foot oil, or sweet lard; I usually put into both a little sheep suet, so make it thick: the way to make each kind is as follows: And first of the oil heating, having by the rules in this book made choice of such herbs, according to their virtues and numbers, which are proper to cure the defect, shred them small and bruise them well in a mortar; then put them into a convenient quantity of oil, imagine to two handfuls of herbs about a pint of oil; if you cannot stay to make it by reason of your present occasions, then set it over the fire, keeping it close covered, and when its near crisp strain forth the oil, and if you desire to make it very strong, then shred more herbs, and bruise them and boil them in the same oil again, until it be crisp, and so strain it, and keep it for your use. But if you desire to make it strong, and have convenient time to do it, then bruise the herbs and put them into the oil, and set them in the Sun for a week or two, then strain it and infuse more herbs, and at length boil them until they be crisp, and having strained it keep it for your use. If you intend to make a cold oil, then infuse the herbs being shred and pounded, as aforesaid, into sweet-lard or neats-feet oil, you may take some of each, and make it after the same manner, as you did the hot oil aforesaid. If these ointments be used about wounds, running sores, or ulcers, then 'twill be convenient to dissolve half an ounce of turpentine in two ounces of oil by the heat of the fire, more especially if you use the hot oil thereunto, otherwise not for every cure, for the most part is antipathetical to the afflicting Planet, except the afflicting Planet be very strong in the heavens, for then you must in some measure comply as I have elsewhere in this book expressed.

Concerning Baths or Fomentations.

Baths are used either case of hot or cold swellings, sometimes for aches, ulcers, wounds, burnings, or scalding, and such like, having by the rules in this book made choice of such herbs and plants, which are necessary for the cure, cut them small and boil them in strong malted water. My usual way is to boil the water and malt together, about three or four pints of malt, to seven or eight pints of water ; when the liquor is strong strain it from the malt and put the herbs into the liquor ; and so soon at it boils take it from the fire ; you must bathe or foment the place grieved warm with the bath, and then immediately use such ointments as are proper for the cure, and so by swath or otherwise according, as the grief is make it up. I commonly use the same herbs in the bath which makes the oil : once a day, being at evening, is my usual time to do it.

Of PURGATIONS.

When you give a Purge, let the *Moon* be in a watery sign, or let a watery sign ascend, and let the *Moon* be aspected by any planet which is direct, if swift in motion and under the earth the better. But by no means let the *Moon* be aspected of any retrograde planet, for then the Patient will be apt to vomit.

Secondly, If you desire to purge any humour, or element predominant, do as follows. Let the planet be weak which is of the nature of the element offending. And let the *Moon* apply to or be in *Trine* or *Sextile* with that planet, which is of contrary

Nature ; as instance Mars, who rules choler, being by nature hot and dry, Now if you desire to purge choler, then let Mars be weak ; and let the Moon be applying to Venus, and if you desire to purge melancholy, which is under ♄; then let ♄ be weak, and the Moon applying to Jupiter : And if you desire to purge flegm let Venus be weak, the Moon decreasing and applying to the Sun by Trine or Sextile aspect : And if to purge blood let Jupiter be weak, and the Moon applying to Mercury : You must do the like in purging any other parts or members of the body, by observing what planet has predominance over it, as instance Saturn rules the spleen, Jupiter rules the liver and lungs, Mars the gall, Sol the heart, Venus the reins and vessels of generation, yet notwithstanding if any planet which owns the infirmity, be Lord of the ascendant of the Patient, and if he be strong its the better, but let the Moon apply by any friendly aspect to a fortune, and if she be in the sign, which represents that part of the body grieved its the better.

Of the manner of purging the Body.

If the body require a strong purge be sure to eat no supper, but if any let it be light of digestion, and take it early before you go to bed. Also before you go to bed take a little aloes in the pap of an apple, so much as will heap on a single penny; but not bruised too small, or otherwise take two or three small pills made suitable to the humour offending : and if the Patient's body be much bound, take either a suppository made with Sal Gem, or a glister to open and prepare the body before the physick works : Take the purge in the morning early, and let the Moon be in a watery sign or else let a watery sign ascend, as is above expressed ; take either water-gruel or thin broth, about an hour after, and likewise after every stool, and fast at least six hours after (I mean from meat) or any other diet.

How to Purge the Head, or remote parts.

When you intend to purge the head or remote parts of the body, you must give the patient pills made up in a hard form, for the longer it remains in the body the better it works upon the remote humours offending.

How to purge Choler.

That which purges Choler gently is peach flowers, blue-violets, damask Roses, centaury : But I chiefly use aloes, and Rhubarb, provided the body be strong, else not.

How to purge Flegm and water.

Elder buds, elder-flowers, broom-flowers, flower-de-luce roots, hyssop, Spurge, dwarf-elder, orris : but I chiefly use bryony root or jallop, the body being strong.

How to purge Melancholy.

Polypodium, fumitory, white and black Hellebore, dodder, Epithymum, Inde Mirabilis, lapis lazuli. But that which I chiefly use is sene and Scammony.

How to purge Blood.

To purge the blood is best done by decoctions made with such herbs, which are suitable to the grief, as you may find elsewhere in this Book ; But if you desire to purge gross humours, proceeding from corruption of blood, as boils, botches, tumors, itches or scabs : Then I commonly use the powder called *pulvus sanctus*, or holy powder, made according to the *London* Dispensatory.

Of Vomits.

When you intend to give a Vomit, let either the *Moon* or Lord of the ascendant be in an earthy sign aspected by a Planet retrograde, and let the sign ascending be an earthy sign, when the vomit is taken ; or let the *Moon* be aspected by planets stationary or slow in motion, if about the earth the better : Any one of these observations will serve where there are no testimonies against it.

Of Baths, or Sweats.

Enter baths or sweats for hot diseases, when the *Moon* is in watery sign, as ♋, ♏, ♓.

Enter baths or sweats, for cold infirmities, when the *Moon* is in fiery signs, as ♈, ♌, ♐.

Of Fluxes, Rheums, and Laxes,

To stay fluxes, Rheums, and Laxes let the *Moon* be in an Earthy sign, as ♑, ♉, ♍.

Of Glisters.

Take Glisters when the *Moon* is in airy or watery signs, especially in ♑ or ♏.

Of Blood-letting.

Let blood on the right side at spring, and on the left-side at the fall.

Blood-letting

Choleric persons must be let blood, when the *Moon* is in watery signs, as ♋, ♏, or ♓.

Phlegmatic persons must be let blood, when the *Moon* is in fiery signs as ♈, ♐, but not in ♌, because that sign governs the heart.

Melancholy persons must be let blood, when the *Moon* is in airy signs, as ♎ and ♒ but not in ♊, because that sign governs the arms, except you let blood in some other part of the body.

Sanguine persons may let blood, when the *Moon* is in any sign except ♌, or the place signified by the sign where the *Moon* is.

Young people may let blood before the first Quarter is over.

Middle age from the first Quarter to the Full.

Elder people from the Full to the last Quarter.

Old people from the last Quarter to the change.

Good to comfort the vertue.	{ Attractive Retentive Digestive Expulsive }	the *Moon* in	{ ♈ ♌ ♐ ♉ ♍ ♑ ♊ ♎ ♒ ♋ ♏ ♓ }

Here follows a Catalogue *of such choice herbs, which cures the most usual infirmities and diseases incident to men and women (being discovered by the* Sun *and* Moon *afflicted in any of the twelve signs, or by a figure of twelve houses) out of which you may make diet drinks, ointments, baths, glisters; fumes, suffumigations, cataplasms, and the like, according to the humour offending : And without question, if rightly understood, may serve to cure all griefs and infirmities whatsoever, although not by me named, as for example, if one shall desire cure for the* Asthma *or shortness of breath, those herbs which open obstructions do it.*

Note, *That all inward griefs or infirmities are usually cured only by decoctions and the spirits of plants, which are extracted from them : And such diseases or infirmities which proceed from the heart and brain, and lie in the nerves and arteries and vital spirits, such as are convulsions, apoplexies, palpitations, palsy ; and such like are not cured only by decoctions, but also by ointments and cataplasms applied to the pulses and other parts suitable : And as concerning all pains, aches, humours, and swellings, baths and ointments, suitable to their condition are most proper : nor omitting diet drinks, corresponding in all cures whatsoever.*

Note, *That I do not use all the herbs named for every Cure, but only a select number, as is elsewhere expressed.*

A

Abortion to hinder : Snakeweed or bistort, madder, moss, sage, tansy, trefoil.

Aches, coming of cold, or taken under cold planets to help : Rosemary, camomile, rue, bayes, Saint *John's* wort, lavender, marjoram, sage, cinquefoil, broom, wormwood, ragwort, mugwort, elmpeel, smallage, comfrey, vervain, wild-tansy, brooklime, arsmart, goutwort, calamint, hyssop, charlock, scabious, southernwood, marigolds.

Aches coming of heat, or taken under *Mars* : Camomile, Saint *John's* wort, balm, arsmart, groundsel, sorrel, archangel, mallows, honeysuckles, violet leaves, elmpeel, elderflowers, comfrey, mugwort, smallage, henbane, chickweed, sea green, turnip, cabbage, cinquefoil, plantain, orpine, daisy, lettuce, spinage, endive, adders-tongue, pimpernel, trefoil, sowthistle.

After-birth and *Secundine* to expel : Angelica, camomile, chervil, horehound, mallows, mugwort, marigolds, pennyroyal, thyme, wake-robin, Alexander, fennel, garlic, housetongue.

Agues, If you intend to cure all kinds of *Agues* you must take notice under what planet the patient is most afflicted, whether under *Saturn* or under *Mars* or both as I have elsewhere expressed in this book, and so make choice of herbs accordingly : Rosemary, lovage, camomile, rue, centaury, southernwood, wood-betony, sage, vervain, feverfew, horsemint, savin, asarabacca, carduus, wormwood, tobacco, burdock, mustard, rhubarb, sorrel, groundsel, plantain, calamint, cinquefoil, fumitory, black hellebore, smallage, satirion, dodder, bryony, agrimony, hyssop, viper's grass, endive, succory, borage, trefoil, periwinkle.

Appetite to procure : Sorrel, sloes, apples, barberries, capers, black-cherries, mulberries, mints, gooseberries, grapes ; generally such herbs, plants, or fruits, which are sour, having no unpleasant relish are good.

Saint Anthony's fire : Rhubarb, rue, saffron, bugloss, brooklime, adders-tongue, houseleek, chickweed, nightshade, white poppy, pondweed, crabtree, danewort, houndstongue, adders-tongue, henbane, lentils, mandrake, hemlock.

Apoplexies : Mistletoe, lavender, wall-gillyflowers, melilot, box, wild citrus, lilly, marjoram, sage, pellitory, fennel, masterwort.

Apostumes : Adders-tongue, bear's breech, melilot, onions, rye, chickweed, daisy, liverwort, privet, vervain, flax, mugwort.

B   B

Back and *Reins* to strengthen : Saint *John's*-wort, balm, angelica, rosemary, mistletoe, clary, mints, cowslips, comfrey, lungwort, borage-blossoms, sweet-maudlin, costmary, mace, *Solomon's*-seal, wood-betony.

Barrenness to help : Barrenwort, clary, Saint *James*-wort, Lady's mantle, herb mercury, horsemint, sage, shepherd's-needle.

Belching for to repress : Aniseed, betony, camomile, marjoram, wormwood, hare's-foot, wood-betony, burnet.

Belly-ache : Camomile, centaury, sweet-marjoram, plantain, smallage, rue, angelica, sage, southernwood, thyme, hyssop, ground-ivy or alehoof, fennel-root, and fennel-seed, fern, stinking gladwin, marshmallows.

Belly to loosen : Basil, bay tree, white-beets, elder-buds, fumitory, houndstongue, laurel, mallows, maidenhair, herb mercury, mirabilan, mulberries, peach flowers, roses, poppy, potatoes, rhubarb, satirion, scabious, sene, spurge, spinach, violet-flowers, leaves, and footstalks.

Belly to bind : Bulleys, caltrop, chestnuts, cowslips, eglantine, Saint *John's*-wort, lentils, ginger, dates, medlars, quinces, rice, services, whortleberries, hot stewed prunes, red-wine.

Bladder to cleanse : Angelica, rosemary, pimpernel, dandelion, borage, burdock, asarabacca, furzbush-flowers, feverfew, chervil, dodder, amphier, southernwood, spignel, vine, white-wine. *Vide, Stone* in the Kidneys, *Reins* and *Bladder*.

Bleeding to stay : Aloe, red-beans, goldenrod, haws, lady's bedstraw, liverwort, moss, archangel, plantain, yarrow, sandalwood, dry dates, chestnuts, comfrey, tormentil, roses, rosemary, burnet, cattail, herb twopence, horsetail, moonwort, mulberries : If the *Bleeding* be at nose, my usual way is to tie the small of the leg and the hand-wrist on that side which bleeds, and to dry some of the patients blood to a powder, and let them snuff it up into their nostrils.

Blood to cleanse : Angelica , rue, sage, scurvy-grass, rhubarb, bloodwort, liverwort, scabious, borage, hyssop, bluebottle, broom-buds, foxgloves, watercresses, elderbuds and berries, burdock, chervil.

Breast and *Stomach* to cleanse : *Vide, Obstructions* to open and remove.

Breath-stinking to help : Rosemary, cowslips, rue, wormwood, balsam, butcher's-broom, smallage, pomecitron, burnet, angelica, sage.

Broken-Bones to help knit : Bugle, elmpeel, butcher's-broom, holly, mastic-tree, self-heal, *Solomon's*-seal, yarrow, bugle.

Burning and *Scalding* to cure : Adders-tongue, asphodel, balm-apple, bear's breech, burdock, chickweed, cattail, coltsfoot, danewort, daffodil, elder, henbane, water-betony, houseleek, lettuce, orpine, plantain, purslane, tobacco, friar's-cowl, cabbage, juice of crabs, or sour apples, sheep's dung.

Burstings or *Ruptures* to cure : Saint *Johns*-wort, comfrey, cinquefoil, *Solomon's*-seal, sanicle, rupturewort, elmpeel, vervain, calamint, yarrow, daisy, goldenrod, knapweed, mouse-ear, valerian, twayblade, adders-tongue, horsetail, balm, century, bugle, juniper, *Venus* wake-robin, *Saturn* twayblade, germander, birthwort, *Saturn* hawkweed, *Saturn* bird's-foot, *Mars* Osmund-royal, *Mars* and water-Osmund.

C   C

Carbuncles to cure : Spurge, tobacco, walnut, vetch, fennel, colewort, or cabbage.

Catarrhs or thin *Rheums* to stay : Saffron, angelica, sweet marjoram, sweet-maudlin, costmary, lavender, Saint-*James* wort, bugloss, calamint, tobacco, spignel, storax.

Child-birth to help : Bugloss, balm-apple, horehound, motherwort, mugwort, parsley, woodbine, sundew, columbine, caraway, cinnamon, parsnip, vine, trefoil, spikenard, mallows, and marshmallows.

Choler and *Phlegm* to purge : Black-alder, aloes, bryony, centaury, elder-buds, endive, fennel, stinking gladdon, black hellebore, hyssop, lungwort, herb mercury, spurge, sycamore, tamarind, tormentil, woad, violet leaves and roots, glasswort, gourds, flower-de-luce, fleawort, Saint *John's* wort, mezereon.

Cholic of wind to ease : Agrimony, aniseed, angelica, apricot, betony, bezar-tree, bryony, camomile, sweet-fennel-seed, coriander-seed, caraway-seed, centaury, cranesbill, daisy, danewort, eglantine, feverfew, galangal, herb true-love, jack by the hedge, lavender, parsley, peach-flowers, horseradish, ribwort, rue, saxifrage, tobacco, tamarisk, zedoary, yarrow, mouse-ear.

Colds, Coughs, and *Hoarseness* to cure : Angelica, pennyroyal, betony, borage, coltsfoot, cinquefoil, clary, horehound, calamint, comfrey, daffodil, elecampane, figs, fennel, germander, stinking gladdon, jack by the hedge, juniper, liquorice, maidenhair, moss, parsley, mouse-ear, rocket, rue, sage, sundew, thyme, tobacco, valerian, vine, zedoary.

Consumptions, to cure : Balsam, barley, cicely, mouse-ear, Jesuit's bark, cullians, melons, moss, vine, burdock, snails, aniseed, arrowhead, borage, bugloss, dandelion, horehound.

Convulsions to cure : Saint *John's* wort, mistletoe, centaury, balm, angelica, clary, mints, cowslips, wood-betony, wallgillyflowers, sage, sweet-marjoram, lavender, southernwood, elecampane, bryony, hawkweed, melilot, wormwood, carduus, garlic, hyssop, asphodel, calamint, danewort, stinking gladdon, heart's ease, sea-holly, sage, thyme, valerian.

Courses of women or monthly terms to provoke : Flower-wort, motherwort, catnip, sage, dill, wood-betony, bayberries, elecampane, herb mercury, wild carrots, hacraper, germander, clary, white-beets, mugwort, stinking gladdon, flower-de-luce, cuckoopint, birthwort, calamint, catmint, feverfew, gillyflowers, gooseberries, groundsel, honeywort, horehound, Saint

John's wort, lovage, pennyroyal, peony, rosemary, rue, saffron, savin, savory, bryony, southernwood, spignel, tansy, wake-robin, wolf's-bane.

Courses of women or the *Reds* to stop : Saint *John's* wort, red beets, red-nettles, arrach, comfrey roots, yarrow, red corral, red pebble-stone, ribwort, coriander, rind of oak, in fume to sit over, juniper, Lady's mantle, lentils, periwinkle, quinces, sanicle, sandalwood, red poppy, tamarisk tree.

Cramps to ease : Asphodel, basil, bear's breech, calamint, wild carrot, elecompane, danewort, flower-de-luce, garlic, sea holly, mistletoe, pennyroyal, rosemary, saffron, southernwood, tobacco, turpentine, vine, woodbine, wolf's-bane, fennel, camomile.

D   D

Deafness to cure : Angelica, bay, balm, lavender, wood-betony, holly, ivy, rue, walnuts, tobacco, hellebore, savory, sene, wormwood, carduus, henbane.

Digestion and *Concoction* to help : Angelica, balm, sweet-marjoram, pennyroyal, spearmint, elecompane, sweet-maudlin, costmary, rocket, tarragon, Jack by the hedge, lovage, radish, camphire, vine, caraway, eglantine, cinnamon, cloves, coriander.

Dogs mad their bitings to cure : Houndstongue, balm, betony, burdock, eglantine, sea-dogs grass, horehound, mugwort, herb mercury, pimpernel, mints, sene, yarrow, box : The flesh of the same dog present cure.

Dropsy to cure : Agrimony, asarabacca, barley, basil, camomile, celandine, centaury, burdock, broom, brooklime, ash, bryony, coffee, dittany, elder, flower-de-luce, garlic, hellebore, box, sea holly, laurel, marjoram, sweet-maudlin, pennyroyal, pimpernel, moss, spurge, tobacco, wormwood, carduus, rosemary, lavender, bayes, rue, smallage, sage, Saint *John*'s wort, hyssop, vervain, tamarisk, rhubarb, saffron, betony, aniseed, parsley.

E   E

Ears pain and noise to help : Jews ears, betony, basil, asphodel, clivers, coriander, danewort, dittany, fennel, hemp-seed, ivy, parsley, pellitory, rhubarb, tamarisk, melilot, bayes, leeks, peach, plantain, marjoram.

Eyesight to quicken : Eye-bright, celandine, white roses, archangel, angelica, balm, centaury, germander, hawkweed, heath, lavender, lovage, elecompane, melilot, meadowsweet, rue, savory, vine, vipers grass, asparagus, wake-robin, valerian.

Eyes inflamed, red or bloodshot to cure : Bluebottle, clary, eye-bright, houseleek, ivy, larkspur, marjoram, meadowsweet, marigold, moss, mullein, plantain, poppy, southernwood, tansy, trefoil, wolf's-bane, yarrow, myrtle, violets, endive.

F   F

Falling-sickness : Peony, mistletoe, rosemary, sweet-marjoram, southernwood, lavender, elecampane, germander, hyssop, wood-betony, sage, costmary, cinquefoil, borage, masterwort, staggerwort, wormwood, carduus, garlic, cowslip, foxgloves, pennyroyal, elder-buds, violets, groundsel, mallows, box, bryony, black cherries, dittany, fennel, rue, hellebore, sea-holly, juniper, laserwort, moss, mouse-ear, purslane, satirion, sene, sundew, thyme, vine, trefoil.

Fevers to cure : Marigolds, roses, hyssop, dandelion, bluebottle, herb twopence, purslane, snakeweed, wormwood.

Fevers burning to cure : Adders-tongue, barley, borage, butterburr, crowfoot, currants, daisies, dandelion, endive, hazeltree, lilly, limes, violets.

Fevers Pestilential, to cure : Angelica, rue, saffron, bishop's weed, carnations, dragons blood, ducks-meat, fluellin, sorrel, scabious, wormwood, sage, burnet, violets.

Flegm to purge : Bryony, butcher's-broom, daffodil, dodder, feverfew, foxgloves, fumitory, stinking gladdon, endive, succory, birthwort, hawkweed, black hellebore, henbane, hyssop, holly-berries, bindweed, allheal, butterwort, elder-buds.

Flowers of women : *See* Courses.

Flux of the belly, and humours to stop : Red beets, bloodwort, box, brambles, bugloss, burnet, cinquefoil, cockshead, cudweed, flower-de-luce, cranesbill, germander, goldenrod, hart's-tongue, holly, horehound, lady's-mantle, moss, orpine, periwinkle, pimpernel, plantain, quince, rice, rupturewort, services, shepherds-purse, spikenard, wormwood.

Flux bloody to stay : Adders-tongue, agrimony, barberries, red beans, bulleys, burnet, chestnuts, cinquefoil, cowslips, prunes, hot dry dates, dock, hazelnuts, herb twopence, holly, rose, houseleek, lilly, madder, maudlin, costmary, meadowsweet, moss, mulberries, oak, oxlips, rosemary, sorrel, whortleberry, yarrow, tormentil, periwinkle, quinces, tansy, self-heal.

French pox to cure : Rue, smallage, hyssop, sea-holly, sage, aloes, marshmallows, southernwood, plantain, damask-roses, asarabacca, cowslip, primrose, hemlock, angelica, wormwood, violet-leaves and flowers, box, danewort, houndstongue, tobacco, tormentil, vipers-grass, hops, vine, tamarisk, dodder, pellitory : There is also two sorts of wood used in diet-drinks, *viz.* Guaicum, and fraxinus, or the gums of them. Note, that in curing this disease, those herbs which are used for baths must be drawing, cleansing, and healing, such as is rue, smallage, hyssop, tobacco, marshmallows, box, eryngo, &c. And the herbs used for diet-drinks must be good to expel poison, purge and cleanse, as rue, aloes, angelica, sage, bayes, cowslips, primrose, plantain, violets, roses; &c. Also the wood or gum called *Guiacum*, and *Fraxinus*. The herbs which makes the oils or ointments must be good to resist poison, cooling and healing, such as rue, angelica, cowslip, damask-roses, plantain, violets, primroses, henbane, hemlock, &c. In this distemper, you must let blood in the neither vein of the yard : by this rule you may cure, if begun in time, but after long continuance in this condition fluxing and other extremities must be used.

Fundament falling to remedy : Snakeweed, galls, blue pimpernel, starwort, cuckoopint, wake-robin.

G   G

Gall, to open : Asarabacca, bugle, calamint, rhubarb, hempseed, bitter-sweet, celandine, centaury, endive, saffron, alehoof, or ground ivy, camomile, dandelion, dodder of thyme or other dodders, quick-grass.

Green-sickness to cure : Asarabacca, broom, centaury, marigolds rhubarbs, maudlin, vine, powder of steel.

Guts stopped, or the iliac passion to cure : Ivy, mints, shepherds-needle, plantain, mallows, southernwood, summer savory.

Gout to cure : See Aches hot and cold.

H   H

Headache to cure, Aloes, basil, betony, bryony, butcher's-broom, cudweed, cumin, dodder, fluellin, frankincense, hellebore, houseleek, ironwort, meadowsweet, melilot, mints, mugwort, moss, nightshade, pennyroyal, spikenard, roses, sycamore, tobacco, thyme, vine, vervain, woodruff.

Headache, to draw to the feet by way of cataplasm : Rue, smallage, bryony, henbane, wormwood, carduus, mallows, lavender, hyssop, hacraper. By this way I cured one Mrs. *Farrell* in *Oxon* a Stationer's wife who was a long time pained after she had tried many others.

Head giddiness and swimmings to cure : Aniseed, catamint, bryony, fennel, bears ears, beets, feverfew, pellitory, pennyroyal, sene, *Solomon's* seal, maudlin, masterwort, olives, saffron, box, thyme, tobacco, wolf's bane, vipers grass, vine.

Head to purge : Celadine, elder-buds, stinking gladdon, laurel, sweet-marjoram, maudlin, costmary, dragons blood, pimpernel, rosemary, sene, sneezewort, *Solomon's* seal, sowbread, clary, vine.

Heart to fortify against infection, and likewise to comfort : Angelica, rosemary, marigolds, balm, borage, bugloss, carnations, saffron, rue, sage, sene, zedoary, motherwort, cinnamon, damask roses, lavender.

Cures: Greensickness to Humours

Hearts fainting or palpitations to cure : Angelica, marigolds, borage, balm, rosemary, bayberries, costmary, burnet, cinnamon, cloves, endive, sage, saffron, nutmeg, strawberries, damask roses, spikenard, galingale, hart's tongue, lavender, sandalwood, vipers grass : Also the hearts of creatures which are good to eat.

Hearing loss to cure : Balm, lavender, bay, bryony, henbane, wood-betony, rocket, southernwood, tobacco, wormwood, rue, carduus, sweet-marjoram, eye-bright, cockshead, turpentine, woodbine.

Hiccups to stay : Birthwort, fennel, hart's tongue, marjoram, shepherd's needle, thyme, skirrets, woodbine, dill.

Hemorrhoids or *piles* to cure : Pilewort, cuckoopint, plantain, wall, pennyroyal, pellitory of the wall, chickweed, catmint, stinking gladdon, goutwort, houndstongue, laurel, leeks, tobacco, lupine, figwort, fig-tree, garlic, vine, fumitory : The root of houndstongue dried under embers in paste or wet paper made into a suppository gives present cure.

Hoarseness, and loss of voice to help : Burdock-root, cherry-tree gum, chervil, cinquefoil, liquorice, horehound, violets, leeks, rosemary, saffron, coltsfoot, turnip, tobacco, lavender.

Humors gross to expel : Aloes, bay, camomile, costmary, calamint, centaury, catmint, foxgloves, fumitory, garlic, hyssop, juniper, lavender, liquorice, mistletoe, motherwort, sage, rue, scurvy-grass, southernwood, sycamore, parsley, heartwort, fennel, nettle, scabious, turbith, vine, horseradish, lovage, spearmint, peach-tree, pennyroyal, Saint *Peter's* wort, polypody of the oak, roses.

I-J

Iliac passion : *See* Guts stopped.

Inflammations to assuage : Apples, barley, beets, bugloss, cleaver, colewort, coltsfoot, endive, succory, gooseberries, hemlock, henbane, horsetail, houseleek, Saint *John's* wort, knotgrass, Lady's mantle, lilly, liquorice, liverwort, melilot, moss, mulberries, nightshade, orpine, pimpernel, purslane, ribwort, sandalwood, *Solomon's* seal, sorrel, sowthistle, violets, wheat, woad, madder, marjoram, cleavers.

Itches to cure : Alehoof or ground ivy, bay, calendine, chickweed, cuckoopint, dock, fumitory, vinegar, hyssop, hops, plantain, roses, cockle, elecompane, mugwort, rhubarb, sene, tobacco, wormwood, vine, stinking gladdon, madder, pondweed.

Jaundies yellow to cure : Aloes, agrimony, the inner yellow bark of black elder, asarabacca, bay, wood-betony, calamint, doder of thyme, flower-de-luce, furzbush flowers, hemp, mouse-ear, hedge-mustard, eryngo and sea-holly, hops, horehound, madder, rosemary, rupturewort, succory roots, wormwood, basil, butcher's broom, bryony, centaury, docks, liverwort, marjoram, roses, rhubarb, rue, saffron, spikenard, tormentil, tamarisk, vine, broom-blossoms, fumitory.

Joints, pained : *See* Aches hot and cold.

K

Kernals and knots in the flesh to cure : Archangel, cinquefoil, mandrake, mugwort, mustard, lupine, pondweed, ribwort, rue, spikenard, tormentil, woad, figwort, white-lilly root.

Kidneys, to cleanse : Kidneywort or wall, pennyroyal, gardentansy, furzbush flowers, dodder, elder, fluellin, hops, juniper, maidenhair, parsley, peony, plantain, fennel, broom-blossoms, southernwood, saxifrage, shepherd's-needle, thyme, spignel.

Kings-Evil to cure : Angelica, bayberries, camomile, balm, burnet, eye-bright, marigold, primrose, costmary, celandine, clary, wood betony, borage, sweet marjoram, archangel, melilot, lavender, bugloss, endive, mistletoe, sorrel, heart's-tongue, foxgloves, pimpernel, southernwood, barley flower or meal, pilewort, rosemary, or the lesser celandine, cleavers, figwort or throatwort, stinking gladdon, burdock, mints, broom-blossoms.

L   L

Lasks or *Looseness* to stay : Agrimony, barberries, bulleys, burnet, chestnuts, cowslips, barley, black-cherries, cinnamon, clivers, darnel, St. *John's* wort, mints, nutmeg, quinces, yarrow, sage, hart's-tongue, furzbush flowers, hazelnuts, filberts, oak, wheat, hot prunes, red wine, red pebbles broke into powder, rupturewort.

Leprosy to cure : Ash-tree bark, bryony, stinking gladdon, black-hellebore, darnel, the melilot flower, calamint, elm-tree bark or leaves, flaxweed, mustard, bay, saffron, tamarinds, thyme, vine, virgins-bower, viper-wine, a snake first roasted with salt, and afterwards burnt and brought into powder of which give the Patient a dram every morning in liquor convenient.

Lethargy or *drowsy evil* to cure : Hogs-fennel, watercress, lavender, mustard, onions, pennyroyal, rosemary, sage, summer savory, Jack by the hedge, thyme, vine.

Liver obstructed, to open and purge : Liverwort, agrimony, dandelion, asarabacca, bay, wood-betony, angelica, celandine, centaury, costmary, daisies, hart's-tongue, dodder, elder buds, camomile, elecompane, broom-blossoms, furzbush-flowers, horehound, hemp, sea-holly, sweet marjoram, plantain, saffron, sorrel, scurvy-grass, sene, tormentil, juniper, liquorice, foxgloves, germander, peach, spicknel, shepherd's-needle, vine.

Lungs to open and cleanse : Lungwort, houndstongue, polypody of the oak, hyssop, Alexander, borage, chervil, cinquefoil, cudweed, horehound, coltsfoot, burdock, vervain, St. *James*-wort, rhubarb, sundew, liquorice, bay, tormentil, angelica, apples, feverfew, sweet marjoram, saffron, sene, dodder, Alexander, birthwort, figs, thyme, vine, rhubarb, zedoary.

M   M

Melancholy to repress and purge : Apples, balsam, angelica, borage, bugloss, elecompane, archangel flowers, cowslips, costmary, burnet, dandelion, feverfew, fumitory, madder, pennyroyal, basil, dodder, frankincense, lavender, saffron, marigolds, thyme, scurvy-grass, tortmentil, sene, vine.

Mirth to cause : Angelica, balm, borage, burnet, carnations, chevril, rosemary, marigolds, saffron, thyme, rose, archangel blossoms, sweet marjoram, also all pleasant fumes.

Mother-fits, suffocation or rising to cure : Motherwort, stinking arrach, balm, bay, burdock, camomile, mugwort, elecompane, spearmint, rosemary, wood-betony, bishop's-weed, burnet, butterburr, caraway, feverfew, masterwort, catmint, pellitory of the wall, peony, summer savory, walnut tree, fennel, germander, Jack by the hedge, juniper, lovage, marigolds, mustard, pennyroyal, rosemary, rhubarb, tobacco, southernwood, spignel, wolf's-bane, vine.

Milk to cause in women's breast : Borage, bugloss, lettuce, vipers, bugloss, barley, cabbage, purslane, rocket, sowthistle, turnip, milkwort, trefoil, anemony, herb-frankincense, Saint *Katharine's* flower, bellflower.

Milk to dry up in women's breast : Asarabacca, basil, red-beans, rue, vine.

Monthly courses : *See* Courses of women.

N   N

Nose bleeding, to stop : *See* Bleeding to stay.

Numbness to remove : Hyssop, lavender bear's-breech, nettles, wormwood, rosemary, clary, chervil, borage, angelica, costmary.

O   O

Obstructions to remove : Angelica, baum, centaury, loveage, rue, rosemary, camomile, Saint *John's* wort, pennyroyal, mints, tansy, costmary, sweet maudlin, wood-betony, endive, succory, dandelion, liverwort, bloodwort, borage, lungwort, hyssop, sage, elder-buds, sweet-marjoram, elecampane, germander, fumitory, rhubarb, saffron, scurvy-grass, vervain, vipers-grass, vine, liquorice, horehound.

Opening plants : Angelica, betony, camomile, calamint, borage, broom, asphodel, bishop's-weed, bay, dandelion, docks, fennel, feverfew, figs, foxgloves, lovage, sea-holly, rose, sage, marigolds, peach, rue, smallage, tarragon, thyme, dragons blood, dropwort, Saint *John's* wort, germander, samphire, radish, roses, dittany, cucumbers, wild citrus, horehound, tamarisk.

P   P

Palsy to cure : Angelica, baum, rosemary, clary, mistletoe, mace, marigolds, borage blossoms, cowslips, sage, camomile, chervil, hyssop, lavender, southernwood, Saint *John's* wort, burnet, bluebottle, feverfew, balsam, bears-ear, box, daffodil, parsnip, sage, summer savory, saxifrage, sene, motherwort, juniper, oxlips, pellitory, pepper, pine, vine, tobacco.

Piles to cure : *See* Hemorrhoids.

Plague or *Pestilence* to cure or prevent : Angelica, baum, celandine, carnations, cicely, colombines, elecampane, dyer's-weed, sage, fumitory, marigolds, snakeweed, one blade, bluebottle, butterburr, chervil or cicely, cinquefoil, cuckoopint, devil's-bit, germander, herb true-love, horehound, ivy, marigolds, pimpernel, rue, scabious, vervain, wheat-meal, Jack by the hedge, juniper, rhubarb, saffron, southernwood, vipers-grass, yarrow, a chick's fundament laid to the *Plague* sore kills the chick and cures the Patient.

Pleurisy to cure : Angelica, chervil, fleawort, lovage, marshmallows, hedge-mustard, scabious, violets, clary, cumin, hawkweed, rhubarb, sage, trefoil, aloes, centaury, Saint *Katherine's* flower, mullein, laserwort, nettle, almonds.

Ptisick to cure : Bilberries, chervil or cicely, costmary, sweet maudlin, knapweed, liquorice, marshmallows, parsley, plantain, polypody of the oak, rosemary, bay, bear's-breech, daffodil, lungwort, mouse-ear, purslane, ribwort, sundew, saffron, masterwort, cranesbill, moss.

Purples to cure : Bishop's-weed, snakeweed, fleawort, purple wort, tormentil, water-germander.

Purging the body of ill humors : Aloes, asarabacca, bryony, box, butterwort, alder tree, danewort, endive, feverfew, laurel, juniper, rhubarb, saffron, tobacco, scabious, spinach, marjoram, swallow-wort, spurge, broom blossoms, saxifrage, turbith, bindweed, herb-terrible, vine.

Q   Q

Quinsey to cure : Cudweed, cinquefoil, lovage, orpine, ragwort, violets, wormwood, calamint, mulberries, vine, broom-blossoms, leeks, madder, rhubarb, Saint *James* wort, danewort.

R   R

Reins, to cleanse : Asparagus roots, sea-holly or eryngo, featherfew, filipendula the roots, hops, saxifrage, succory, tansy, grasie, pellitory, pimpernel, rhubarb, herb mercury.

Running of the *Reins* to cure : Blites, liverwort, dock, aromatical reed, rupturewort, *Solomon's*-seal, spleenwort, artichokes, apples, comfrey, dandelion, sea-holly, bear's-foot, sanicle, *Venus* turpentine, snakeweed, yarrow, flower-de-luce, knotgrass, sandalwood, red-roses, amber and *Venus* turpentine given with the white of an egg roasted morning and evening cures, *Probatum*.

Rheums, to stay : Costmary, sweet-maudlin, sciatica-cresses, knot-grass, dog's-mercury, nep or catmint, plantain, red-roses, sage, bay, bugloss houndstongue, hazelnuts, aromatical reed, coriander.

Rest to procure : *See sleep.*

Rickets : Ashen-keys, coffee. Herbs which are good to open obstructions, and are cleansing, strengthening and cordial, being made into ointments and diet drinks will cure.

Ringworms : Bayberries, borage, bugloss, celandine, hemlock, hops, sengreen, liverwort, dog's-mercury, plantain, rue, scabious, sorrel, oil of wheat, alcanet, garlic, hellebore, vine.

Ruptures : *See* Burstings.

S   S

Scabs and *Scurfs* to heal : Alehoof or ground ivy, black alder tree, ash-tree bark, bay, barberries, beets, wood-betony, bryony, bugle, burdock, clary, sciatica-cresses, dock, flaxweed, foxgloves, goldenrod, hops, horehound, cow-parsnip, pellitory of the wall, agrimony, catmint, fumitory, scabious, savin, sene, tobacco, spurge, dodder, elecompane, beech, beets, bloodwort.

Scaldings to cure : *See* Burnings.

For a *Scald head* the bark of ash-tree burnt to ashes, and made into a lye to bath withal cures, *probatum est.*

Sciatica or *hip gout* to cure : Alehoof or ground-ivy, angelica, archangel, asparagus, burdock, cinquefoil, sciatica-cresses, dock, flaxweed, fumitory, stinking gladwin, groundsel, henbane, St. John's wort, kidneywort, or wall, pennyroyal, mustard, nettles, the white poplar, ragwort, wild-tansy, asarabacca, broom, lesser centaury, goutwort, Jack by the hedge, madder, rue, southernwood, tobacco, thyme, trefoil, laserwort, mallows.

Serpents stingings, or *venomous bitings*, to cure : Adders-tongue, Alexander, asarabacca, calamint, elecompane, fern, asphodel, betony, bugloss, hart's-tongue, sea-holly, horehound, houseleek, madder, moss, nettles, peony, bayes, rue, scabious, sperage, sycamore, trefoil, wolf's-bane, burdock, cudweed, germander, scorpion-grass.

Spleens, diseases, obstructions, and *inward swellings* to cure : Alehoof or ground-ivy, Alexander, archangel, asarabacca, baum, bay tree, beets, wood-betony , calamint, camomile, centaury, dandelion, water-fern, furzbush-flowers, germander, stinking gladwin, hart's tongue, hawkweed, hops, horehound, ivy, lavender, broom-flowers, marshmallows, mistletoe, mustard, horseradish, southernwood, lady's thistle, tormentil, winter-gillyflowers, woad, marjoram, rocket, tamarisk, thyme, vervain, wormwood, dittander, dodder of thyme, angelica, rhubarb, scurvy grass, spleen-tree, fumitory, sene, rosemary, peach-flowers, parsley, samphire, elder-buds.

Stomach bad to help cleanse strength : Agrimony, apples, avens, bay tree, wood-betony, chervil, costmary, sweet-maudlin, crosswort, endive, elecompane, flower-de-luce, hawkweed, houndstongue, peach-flowers or leaves, dock bastard, rhubarb, the seed or root, sorrel, currants, angelica, baum, Alexander, sweet-marjoram, quinces, capers, succory, dandelion, dodder, Jack by the hedge, liquorice, lovage, mints, moss, young charlock, mustard, tansy, thyme, wormwood, roses, scurvy grass, horseradish, vine, camomile, pennyroyal, gooseberries, purslane, spinage, lettuce, oranges, strawberries, moss, vine, walnuts, myrobalans, fennel, rue, spignel, limes, Saint *John's* wort.

Stitches or side-pains to ease : Avens, wood-betony, bryony, camomile, wild-carrots, parsley, sage, our lady's thistle, garden valerian, asphodel, birthwort, chervil, elecampane, camomile, fennel, germander, larkspur, melilot, mistletoe, rupturewort, stitchwort, trefoil, thyme, rue, vine.

For the S T O N E : Saxifrage, pellitory of the wall, mother of thyme, parsley, radishes, stilled out of milk in a cold still.

Stone and *Gravel* to expel : Apples, apricot, bean, bramble, brooklime, broom blossoms, furzbush flowers, betony, dandelion, bay tree, burdock, camomile, carnations, adonis flower, wild carrots, black-cherries, colombine, cockle, cowslips, feverfew, sorrel, mugwort, pimpernel, cranesbill, dittany, dodder, dropwort, eglantine, fennel, goldenrod, couchgrass, haws, Jack by the hedge, Saint *James* wort, Saint *John's* wort, lady's bedstraw, liverwort, marshmallows, masterwort, maidenhair, medlar-stones, melilot, mints, moss, nettle, nutmeg, ox-eye, parsley, parsnip, pellitory, pennyroyal, periwinkle, peony, purslane, violet, radish, rhubarb, spignel, tansy, thyme, vervain, wolf's-bane, trefoil, vine.

Stone in the *Kidneys* and *Reins* to expel : Aromatical reed, balsam, beech, birch-tree, bramble, cabbage, danewort, goldenrod, maidenhair, parsley, pennyroyal, rupturewort, saxifrage, dandelion, furzbush flowers, strawberries, medlar-stone, young turnip-leaves, butcher's-broom, broom, groundsel.

Cures: Stiches to Spots 103

Strangury or *Pissing* stopped to help : Agrimony, angelica, Alexander, rosemary, pimpernel, apples, basil, betony, brooklime, dandelion, daisies, broom, sweet marjoram, asarabacca, butcher's-broom, feverfew, fennel-root, borage, bramble, liquorice, centaury, dittany of Crete, dropwort, eglantine, germander, stinking gladwin, couch-grass, gromwell, hawkweed, hops, horsetail, juniper, larkspur, herb mercury, mints, pellitory, spikenard, radish, saxifrage, southernwood, tansy, thyme, tormentil, trefoil, valerian, vine, groundsel.

Swellings : See Aches hot and cold.

Swoonings and *Faintings* to cure : Aromatical reed, basil, borage, balm, dodder of thyme, motherwort, sweet marjoram, pennyroyal, rosemary, angelica, sundew, vine, cinnamon, endive, costmary, tobacco, vine, viper's-grass, quinces, cherries.

Sinews shrinking to help : Camomile, chickweed, elmpeel, comfrey, oil of trotters, hog's-fennel, laserwort, turpentine, oil of young puppies under nine days old.

Sinews, to strengthen : Balsam, centaury, cowslip, fennel, flower-de-luce, Lady's bedstraw, mints, rosemary, sage, pellitory, yarrow, tansy, Saint John's wort.

Spitting of blood to stay : Clowns-all heal, borage, comfrey, dock, elecompane, Saint John's wort, inner bark of oak, plantain, sage, betony, fennel, hart's tongue, red beets, red archangel, leeks, lungwort, bramble, moss, purslane, ribwort, sanickle, trefoil, bloodwort, rhubarb, shepherds-purse, arrowhead, barberries, almonds, horehound, holly, rose.

Spots, *Freckles*, and *Pimples* in the skin to clear : Basil, bayes, bell-flower, broom blossoms, bryony, elecompane, feverfew, fumitory, roses, calamint, celandine, coleworts, daffodil, dittander, endive, flower-de-luce, hawkweed, lovage, onions, parsley, pennyroyal, radish, rocket, rosemary, savin, scurvy grass, *Solomon's* seal, strawberries, tansy, vervain, wheat.

Sleep to procure : Anet, barley, cowslips, endive, lettuce, saffron, white poppy, purslane, roses, sensitive herbs, tobacco, virgins-bower, wormwood, henbane, hemlock, lilly, parsley, nightshade, nutmeg, onions, herb true-love, vine, mandrake, moss, dandelion, ploughman's-spikenard, stinking gladwin.

Scurvy to cure : Brooklime, watercresses, horseradish, cuckoo flower, danewort, juniper, scurvy-grass, horsetail, fluellin, vine, wayfaring-tree, tamarinds, cloudberries, coffee.

Shingles to cure : Cinquefoil, houseleek, rue, pellitory, olive-tree, *Egyptian*-thorn, lentil, cow, parsnip, plantain.

Surfeits to cure : Angelica, coleworts, liverwort, wormwood, broom-blossoms, red poppy, saffron, violets, red roses, clove-gillyflowers, aniseed, coliander, figs, raisins.

T T

Terms : *See* Courses.

Tetters to heal : Beech-tree, celandine, hops, horehound, liverwort, plantain, sorrel, oil of green wheat, darnel, alcanet, almonds, cresses, fluellin, jessamine, hellebore, St. *James*-wort, limes, myrtle, pine, rhubarb, swallow-wort, vine.

Throat-Almonds to help : Dill, boxthorn, bramble, cedar, cinquefoil, devil's-bit, caltrops, elder, fumitory, mustard, pellitory, primrose, smallage.

Throats kernels and *swellings* to waste : Sorrel, blackthorn leaves, alder, clivers, fumitory, hyssop, St. James-wort, orach, plums, rampions, rhubarb, snakeweed, starwort, throatwort, or bell flowers, camomile.

Throat-soreness and *Diseases* to help : Ground-ivy, pellitory of the wall, red-roses, sage, self-heal, blackthorn leaves, vine-leaves, elder-flowers, barley, bulleys, columbine, fig-tree, hyssop, toadstools, woodbine, goldenrod, camomile.

Throats Inflammation to assuage : Cuckoopint root, walnut-tree, strawberries, throatwort, toadstools, vine-leaves, violets, wormwood, camomile.

Toothache, to help : Black alder, arsmart root or seed, asparagus root, red beet-root, broom, ivy-berries, broom-rape, cinque-foil-roots, flower-de-luce roots, pennyroyal, tamarisk-tree, angelica, asphodel, basil, box, burdock, cammock, celandine, crowfoot, toothwort, henbane, hemlock, mustard, nettles, pellitory, poppy, pockweed, rhubarb, saffron, spurge, sundew, tobacco, tamarisk, vervain, wormwood, yarrow, hyssop.

U-V   U-V

Ulcers and *sores* to heal : Agrimony, black-alder, allheal, aloes, angelica, balsam, barley, betony, birthwort, bugle, bryony, broom-blossoms, bramble, centaury, clary, butterburr, campion, clivers, cockle, coltsfoot, coleworts, comfrey, dandelion, dodder, elder-blossoms, elecompane, cudweed, wintercresses, foxgloves, ground-pine, goat's-beard, gourds, germander, heart's-ease, herb true-love, hellebore, henbane, horehound, mistletoe, pimpernel, sage, savin, St. *John's*-wort, juniper, hyssop, houndstongue, masterwort, cudweed, holly, rose, lilly, mullein, pondweed, plantain, pine, rhubarb, poppy, roses-red, smallage, snakeweed southernwood, self-heal, valerian, wake-robin or cuckoopint, zedoary, yarrow, lentils, bears-ears.

Ulcers or *sores* running and spreading to cure : Adders-tongue, anemony, arsmart, asphodels, endive, *Egyptian* thorn, darnel, dodder, camels-hay, celandine, crosswort, dragons blood, figwort, fluellin, friar's-cowl, bears-ears, holly, rose, hemlock, Jack by the hedge, hops, horse-tongue, houseleek, ivy, knapweed, meadowsweet, moss, oats, oil-pulse, olive-tree, pondweed, rose-wood, smallage, tobacco, tamarisk-wood, wolf's-bane, vetch, foxstones, cinquefoil, bluebottle, red wild campions.

Ulcers–hollow, and *Fistulas* to cleanse : St. *James* wort, hellebore, houndstongue, fox-stones, friar's-cowl, spurge, knapweed, juniper, ivy, plantain, ribwort, tormentil, vervain, yarrow, wintergreen, wound-tree.

Ulcers hollow to fill with flesh : Honeywort, frankincense, lentils, maudlin, costmary, pitch, thorow-wax, juniper.

Ulcers in the privy parts to cure : Apples, avens, baum, bramble, bugle, cranesbill, plantain, cresses, ducks-meat, fenugreek, goldenrod, holly, rose, knotgrass, lungwort, sage, tansy, woodbine, throatwort, galingale, privet.

Urine to Provoke : Alexanders, aniseed, apples, aromatical reed, artichoke, asarabacca, asphodel, basil, bayes, white-beets, bramble, bryony, burdock, butchers-broom, calamint, cedar, bear's-breech, caraways, carrots, black-cherries, chervil, cockshead, coriander, crabs, watercresses, dodder, dragons blood, dandelion, dropwort, dyer's-weed, elecampane, endive, fennel, fluellin, fumitory, furzbush flowers, galingale, garlic, germander, stinking gladdon, goldenrod, gooseberries, hartwort, herb twopence, sea-holly, hops, horse-tongue, Jews-thorn, Saint *John's* wort, juniper, ivy, knotgrass, lavender, laurel, leeks, liverwort, lovage, lupine, madder, sweet-marjoram, masterwort, maudline, costmary, medlars, maidenhair, melilot, herb mercury, millet, moss, myrtle, nettle, oak, onions, parsley, parsnip, pellitory, pennyroyal, periwinkle, radish, polypody, rocket, rosemary, rhubarb, rue, saffron, sage, samphire, savin, scabious, shepherd's needle, smallage, southernwood, spikenard, tarragon, thyme, trefoil, valerian, woodbine, vine.

Vertigo : *See* Heads–giddiness.

Venomous beasts, or *Vipers-biting* to cure : Ash-tree, sweet basil, white beets, borage, burdock, cabbage, century, danewort, or dwarf-elder, elecompane, flower-de-luce, hart's-tongue, houndstongue, hyssop, horehound, St. *John's* wort, knotgrass, mustard, pennyroyal, cliver, woad, or dyer's-weed, wormwood, scorpion-grass, juniper, viper's-grass, woundwort, yew, trefoil.

Vomiting to repress : Spearmint, crabs, onions, adders-tongue, cinnamon, ash keys, cranesbill, currants, fennel, couch grass, *Egyptian* thorn, lady's mantle, liverwort, marjoram, mastic-tree, myrobalans, moonwort, moss, pennyroyal, purslane, quinces, *Solomon's* seal, snakeweed, tormentil, trefoil, whortleberries, wormwood, zedoary, vine.

Vulva fallen to help : Columbine, dittany, hart's-tongue, mouse-ear, mulberries, primrose, cowslips, cuckoopint, or wake-robin.

W W

Wind to expel : Angelica, Alexanders, aniseed, bay tree, dill, elecampane, balsam, birthwort, bryony, camomile, feverfew, fennel, masterwort, melilot, caraways, catmint, cinnamon, coffee, cumin, dragons blood, mints, oats, parsley, elder-buds, galingale, garlic, ginger, hemp seed, holly, rose, hyssop, juniper, ivy, loveage, Jack by the hedge, winter and summer savory, valerian, walnuts, nutmeg, pepper, pockweed, red poppy, rosemary, rue, saffron, sage, tobacco, tansy, thyme, toothwort, wormwood, motherwort, zedoary, vine, tamarisk.

Whites or reds to stay : Agrimony, adders-tongue, red-beets, red archangel, snakeweed, cinquefoil, comfrey, liverwort, red roses, myrtle, oak, *rosa solis* or sundew, rosemary flowers.

Womb to open and cleanse : Angelica, bishop's-weed, balsam, betony, birch-tree, birthwort, bryony, feverfew, butcher's-broom, camomile, fennel, figs, flower-de-luce, lavender, dog's-mercury, mandrake, rue, mouse-ear, savin, vine.

Worms to kill : Agrimony, aloes, arrowhead, arsmart, sweet-apples, pearmain and pippin, butterburr, celandine, devil's-bit, box, calamint, century, ivy-berries, onions, danewort, horseradish, wormwood, garlic, wormseed, feverfew, eglantine, elecampane, fern, gall of an ox, hazel-tree, hemp, henbane, hops, horehound, hyssop, juniper, lavender, sweet-maudlin, mustard, rocket, rhubarb, southernwood, tobacco, tansy, thyme, vervain, walnut-tree, wolf's-bane, zedoary. Make a plaster with wormwood, garlic, celandine, feverfew, and mints, stamped together with the gall of an ox and vinegar ; apply this plasterwise to the belly, and it will both kill and bring forth the worms.

Wounds green to help : Adders-tongue, agrimony, wood-betony, bird's-foot, bluebottle, allheal, arsmart, broom, bugloss, celandine, cranesbill, dyer's-weed, elecampane, elm, plantain, bugle, burnet, fluellin, foxgloves, herb true-love, hyssop, Saint *James* wort, Saint *John's* wort, lungwort, melilot, mallows, moss, orpine, self-heal, sensitive herb, tobacco, yarrow, shepherd's-purse, trefoil, clowns woundwort, comfrey, cudweed, sanicle, devil's-bit, fern, figwort or throatwort, houndstongue, loosestrife, pear tree.

Wounds, inflammations to assuage : Adders-tongue, chickweed, daisy, horehound, loosestrife, one blade, strawberries, vervain, yarrow, balm-apple, houseleek, soapwort, primrose, orpine, purslane.

Wounds to heal : Asarabacca, balm-apple, balsam, baum, bears-ears, adders-tongue, birds-eye, bluebottle, arsmart, bugle, bugloss, burnet, cranesbill, crosswort, daisy, fern, elder-buds or flowers, goldenrod, herb two-pence, bears-ears, horehound, Saint *John's* wort, ivy, houndstongue, loosestrife, lungwort, madder, mastic, maudlin, costmary, moonwort, oak, plantain, rue, sanicle, self heal, satirion, *Solomon's* seal, southernwood, sundew or *rosa solis*, tormentil, turpentine, valerian, twayblade, woad, yarrow, zedoary, woodruff, tobacco, lady's mantle, clowns-wound wort, foxgloves, hyssop.

Y   Y

Yellow Jaundies, *See* Jaundies

Here follows some examples of such griefs and infirmities which were by the Rules aforesaid both Astrologically Discovered and Cured.

I shall relate only two Cures done at *Oxon* : I could have inserted many more done within that City during the time of my abode there, but I am unwilling over-much to enlarge my Book, or trouble the Reader therewith ; these two being enough for satisfaction.

I cured the Daughter of Mr. *Brown* living in *High-street* in *Oxon*, Anno 1658. This was the first cure I did within that City : This Maid having been about Twelve months under the Cure of several *Doctors*, and her Father finding that her grief rather increased than diminished, and hearing by some what great Cures I had done in other places, came to me, and after some communication I erected a Figure, by which, according to the rules of *Astrology* I quickly found what was the Distemper and the cause thereof ; which I am confident no Drug-*Doctor* could do by the Urine : her grief proceeding from an extraordinary distemper of the heart and brain, and not without some rising in the throat by Flegm, and ill Matter settled between Throat and Stomach ; her condition for the time being, was as follows ; She had near a dozen fits a day, which took her somewhat like the falling-sickness but mixed with Convulsion, for during the time of her fit, she seemed senseless with some small striving, and so revived again but not without some sighing and sadness : She was afflicted under the *Sun* and *Mercury*, the one having predominancy over the heart, the other the brain, and so by consequence the Nerves and Arteries oppressed ; the one causing deadness, the other senselessness for the time being of her fit : I judged it to be one kind of Evil, which would

Cure in Oxon: Sun and Mercury Oppressed 111

without question (if not cured) have turned to that which is usually called the *Kings-Evil* ; for in length of time when the Nerves are oppressed, it many times causes white kernels, swellings sometimes in the Throat, and at other times in the Eyes, and indeed in any part of the body, more especially in that part signified by the Sign wherein the principle significator of the sick is afflicted, and then, but not before it's usually called the *Kings Evil* : The way of cure, was as follows in the first place I gave her three solary herbs to wear about her, having a virtue agreeing with the nature of Gold and serves instead of Gold, for as Gold is under the dominion of the *Sun* as being a Metal, so likewise are many herbs and plants under the dominion of the *Sun* accordingly as being vegetable, and being gathered at the right Planetary hours according to their number works the same effects in cure, being worn or otherwise. This cure was effected by such herbs suitable to the grief which were by antipathy to *Mercury*, a Planet cold and dry, *viz.* under *Jupiter*, a Planet hot and moist, but by herbs which were by sympathy, under the *Sun*, for let the *Sun* be strong or weak there it no opposing of him, as being fountain of life ; for in all cures whatsoever, herbs of the *Sun* must be used, and the rather in this cure, by reason the Maid was by nature Melancholy, and likewise afflicted under *Mercury* a Melancholy Planet. In all kinds of *Evils*, the plants and herbs used for cure, must be gathered at the right Planetary hours according to their virtues and numbers : had this Maid been by nature Choleric, then we might have used herbs under *Venus*, or the *Moon*, as being afflicted under the *Sun*, for in all cures we must help to support Nature's defects, so well, as to fortify the Heart ; but most usually Melancholy People are afflicted under Melancholy cold Planets : and Choleric People under hot planets, more especially in *Evils*, for every Element Naturally sympathizes with its own like, and does more vehemently strike thereupon than on the contrary, even as the actions of Men and Women naturally sympathize with their Complexions be it Choler, or Melancholy, *&c.*

Another Cure done in Oxon on the Daughter of Mr. Collins, a Baker, Anno 1669.

THis Maid for some time was troubled with Convulsion-fits, now her Parents being willing to have remedy, went to several *Doctors*, and others for remedy, who used such Physical means, and other remedies as they thought meet : at length they used hot baths wherein they shrank up both her legs, after which, not knowing what more to do for her, they willingly left the Cure ; by which it appeared, that the remedy was worse than the disease ; for instead of curing her distemper, they left her limbs useless ; whereupon, hearing of me, and the many great cures which I had done for others, they came to me desiring to know, whether I could help her distemper, and cure her limbs ? For as they said, having spent much money upon her already, they would not willingly part with any more, except I would undertake to perfect the Cure : After some discourse, having taken an exact time whereby to erect my Figure, and finding that it was Radical by the rules of Astrology, I found that the Maid was curable ; whereupon, having agreed with them for the Cure, at a price, provided if I did not perfect the cure, I was to lose both my charges and pains : I made entrance thereupon, and within some short time I did (through God's blessing) recover both her heath and Limbs, and she has so continued ever since. By the Figure, I found that the *Moon* and *Mercury* were Principally concerned, as having the greatest Predominancy over her distemper, the one ruling over the bulk of the brain, the other over the acting and sensitive part of motion, and so between them making her fits violent and strong : Those afflicting Planets having relation to the Twelfth House, (and no Fortune or Lord of the Tenth House, interposing), gave strong suspicion of an Evil upon the Maid, neither in my opinion was it otherwise : and that was one

Second Cure in Oxon: Moon and Mercury

great reason why the *Doctors* and others could not help her ; for Evils are of that nature that except they be cured by the rules of *Astrology* (without a Miracle) they are seldom, or never cured, for the more they are tampered with, the worse commonly they will be ; for in this condition those herbs and plants which are used, must be gathered at the right Planetary hours, and according to their Numbers, Elemental Qualities, and Virtues, as I have elsewhere expressed ; the manner of cure was as follows, *First*, having gotten three solary Plants which were gathered at the hour of the *Sun*, I gave them the Maid to wear about her Neck instead of Gold, for as Gold is a Metal under the *Sun*, and has a strong virtue to withstand the Evil, so likewise such herbs which are under the *Sun* are approved to have the same virtue accordingly, being gathered as aforesaid. *Secondly* I made choice of such herbs and plants which were Antipathetical to the *Moon* and *Mercury* and so to oppose *Mercury*, I took herbs under the Dominion of *Jupiter* a Planet hot and moist, whereas *Mercury* is cold and dry and to oppose the *Moon*, a Planet cold and moist, I took herbs under *Mars* and the *Sun* both hot and dry out of which herbs being collected according to their Numbers, Elemental Qualities and Virtues, and gathered at the right Planetary hours : I made Diet-drinks, Oils, and Cataplasms. The manner how to make them I have shown elsewhere in this Book : only to the Oil applied to her Legs, I mixed it with oil of young Puppies under nine days old, and with the jelly of Calves Legs which did help cause the sinews being shrunk to extend and stretch forth : after I had used this oil about nine days, having gotten good help, we stretched forth her Legs ; and did split them fast, and about a week after she assayed to move with Crutches, after which continuing the ointment, and keeping her Legs splitted in some short time being young she recovered : also by Diet-drinks & applying Cataplasms to the hand-wrists, not omitting Planetary oils, applied to the heart and brain made out of those herbs collected as aforesaid, she was likewise recovered of her Convulsion Fits, but against the good will and liking of those who had her formerly in cure, and some others their partakers, for it seems they were so troubled about the cure by reason they could not do it, that they made the *Vice Chancellour* acquainted therewith, pretending that I had cured this Maid by unlawful means ; whereupon, Mr. *Collins* this Maid's Father was sent for, to give him account concerning the way and means used for his daughter's cure, who it seems gave him such ample satisfaction therein, that I never was much troubled more ; only the said *Chancellour* sent two Scholars to dispute with me, the one was, as I was informed a Doctor, the other a Master of Arts who after two or three hours discourse, were fully satisfied concerning the Legality of my Art and Profession and as they told me at parting, they did believe, I should have no more trouble therein, yet notwithstanding, those who were my adversaries would not rest contented, but did on the Sabbath day put up Bills to the Ministers to Pray and Preach against me, and my Art ; which when I understood, I could not forbear to smile, remembering a pretty story of a rich Usurer who lived in *London.* A Friend of his desired him to go with him [to] hear a Sermon, the Preacher having notice of his coming spoke much against Usury and Usurers, and all those that went to them ; whereupon, the Sermon being ended, the Usurer's Friend asked him how he liked the Sermon, he said very well, and wished there more such Preachers, why said his friend? To speak against you, and all those of your Profession ? I care not for that said the Usurer, for the more its cried down and the fewer there be of my Profession, the more custom I shall have ; for the Usurer was resolved Preach what they could against it, never to give over his Trade. And the truth is, after the Ministers had Preached against me and my art, I had twice so much custom as I had before, for they could not have done me better service, for many which before had not heard of me made much enquiring after me, hearing what great cures I had done. Not long after came two men who warned me to depart by a day, pretending they had order, I was informed they were *Apothecaries* however to avoid trouble, in regard I was no graduate Doctor, nor yet free of the City, I thought it best to depart and live where I formerly had done in the Parish of *Aldermaston* near *Reading* : but the Citizens never left me, for to this day, I have many cures out of the City, and places near adjoining not withstanding I live ten miles distant. Would I have been at the charge of a License I would have lived there in spite of all my adversaries, but I am well pleased to live where I am having practice enough.

One Cure lately done in Berkshire, Anno. 1667.

One Mr. *Peter Wickens*, living in the Parish of *Tilehurst*, in the County of *Berks*, having lain Bedridden for some time past, who could wag neither hands nor legs, he made trial of many Physicians, Mountebanks and others, but could find no help, continuing rather worse than any whit amending : at length he sent to me, for as I have already declared, I am seldom employed but in case of great necessity (the reasons I have shown elsewhere) ; and having by the rules of *Astrology* discovered the grief with its cause and termination : I undertook the cure at a price, and performed the same in about eight weeks time, he has been since at *London* and has gone several other journeys, and has continued well to this present time of my writing hereof : The cure was performed as follows, Having by the rules of *Astrology* discovered *Saturn* to be the afflicting Planet who was both weak and peregrine, I effected the cure by antipathy, *viz.* by herbs under the dominion of *Jupiter*, and *Sol* ; what herbs are good for *dead-Palsies* I have set down elsewhere in this book, and likewise under what Planet each herb is governed out of which having collected a select number agreeing to each Planet by the rules before going : I made both Oils, Cataplasms, and

Diet-drinks; with the Oils we anointed the brain, reins of his back, cliches [clinches?] of his arms, groin, knees, and ankles, together with heart and stomach. The Cataplasms we applied to the feet, and hand-wrists. The Diet-drink I ordered him to take three times a day, *viz.* morning, and after dinner, and at night. I also ordered him to take Water-gruel made with herbs suitable to his condition every morning, about an hour after he had taken the Diet-drinks ; sometimes in this infirmity we use suffumigations to the head more especially when we find the Patient under a cold dryness : also the diet and food which they eat who are in this condition must be nutritive and of easy digestion ; the Patients in this condition will be very apt to be bound in their body, not only for want of exercise, but also by reason the applications are for the most part hot, wherefore sometimes we give them Glisters, Pills, or Suppositories according to discretion.

The King's Evil

Here follows the way Astrologically not only to discover but also to cure all sorts of Evils, *together with that commonly called, the* Kings-Evils.

Concerning the Evil *commonly called the* Kings-Evil, *and the Cure thereof as follows.*

IT'S generally called the *Kings-Evil*, in regard it pleased God to give the Kings of this Nation that great gift of curing these kinds of infirmities : 'Tis not as many foolishly imagine, called the *Kings-Evil* in regard of any sins by them committed, and so for that cause it should fall upon the Subject : for the *Evil* is directly from themselves occasioned by some extraordinary distemper of the brain, and so from thence dispersed by the Nerves into several parts of the body sometimes I have known it fall into the Eyes, and at other times into the Neck and Throat with white kernels, swellings ; and sometimes 'twill be in any other parts of the body and the swelling is always white. Now in regard that Surgeons and Doctors in former times were ignorant, not only of the Cause but also of the way of cure by reason it lay wholly in the Nerves, for these kinds of *Evils* coming wholly from the Brain as aforesaid : at the first beginning never touches upon the Flesh, Brain, or Blood only the Nerves are puffed up and rise in kernels white, whereupon such applications which usually cured other swellings were clear antipathetical to these kinds of swellings, and rather increased than any way diminished their pain : I have cured many of this kind of *Evil* also, as is well known to many in the Country. Many times it falls out to be in the *Optic* Nerves, and then the Eyes are in a very sad condition. About a year ago I cured the Daughter of one *John Alexander*, living in *Mortimer* in the County of *Berks*, she was taken in both Eyes, they were so closed up, that she could not endure to have them opened whereby to apply any remedy, she lay thus above six months quite blind, besides what time the grief was drawing on before, and the more they tampered with her the worse she was ; at length they were fearful that her Eyes would perish in her head, (as it seems one Maid did who was of their acquaintance). Whereupon they came to me and having agreed upon the price for the cure, I undertake and performed it in about a month's space ; the manner how I performed it I shall relate before I conclude, I find that in former ages multitudes perished through these kinds of Evils, by reason (as I said before) that Doctors and Surgeons were ignorant of the true cause of the distemper, and so by consequence of the cure ; whereupon it pleased God to give this gift of healing, first, to King *Edward* who for his piety was called the Confessor, who was the first *English* King, who succeeded after the *Danes* were extinguished, and after him successively this great gift has continued to the Kings of this Nation : I shall now proceed to set forth the way of cure, not only of this man's Daughter in question, but also how to cure it in any part of the body, provided it be taken in hand in time, before the Nerves, Flesh and Bones are perished, for in length of time, if it be not cured, 'twill get into the Flesh, Bones, and Blood : and then in the end, commonly that Limb or Member of the Body, be it arm, foot, leg, and sometimes thigh and all is cut off : The way of curing this Maid's eye, was as follows. In the first place I made choice of three solary herbs which are esteemed good for the Nerves *viz*, rosemary, Angelica, and balm, these herbs I caused to be made close up in a linen cloth (taking a small quantity of each, being all gathered at the hour of the *Sun*) and gave it her to wear about her Neck instead of Gold, for as Gold is a Metal under the Dominion of the *Sun*, and has a virtue to comfort the brain ; for the Sun has predominancy over the brain, as I have shown elsewhere : see also these herbs being under the Dominion of the *Sun* has the like sympathetic virtue to comfort the brain : accordingly also I made choice of a select number of solary herbs to make a Diet-drink by way of decoction ; and likewise to make an oil to anoint the brain. But to the Eyes I applied only Celandine-water, given in a small tincture of *Roman*-Vitriol ; but at the first beginning of the Cure, I did for a few days apply raw-fresh meat to the powl or Neck to help dry and divert the humour from the Eyes ; by this means through God's blessing she was soon recovered. Now the way to cure this kind of Evil when it settles in any other part of the body, is as follows, You must in the first place make use of three Solary Herbs, as aforesaid, to wear about their neck : also you must make a bath of Solary Herbs, according to the number before mentioned, belonging to the *Sun*, and being gathered at the right Planetary hour : also out of the same herbs, you must make an ointment, and once a day you must bath the place grieved pretty hot, and then immediately with this ointment anoint it, and keep it moderately warm, you must be sure to make choice of such solary herbs, which are esteemed good for the brain and nerves, as you will find in this Book elsewhere : I shall relate one *Example*, This year I cured a Maid, who was the only daughter of Mr. *Henry Bulstrode*, living in *Warfield* Parish in the County of *Berks*, she had the evil in her ear and right side of her head, being most grievously pained therewith : Her Father tried many Doctors and others to his great cost and charge, but instead of mending she grew worse every day than other, and the more they tampered with her ; the more she was afflicted ; the swelling was white, she was in this condition about nine months : at length finding no remedy, and hearing by some of his Neighbours, what great cures I had done for others, her Father came to me, and having agreed with me about the charge, I undertook the cure, and in about six weeks time did perfect the cure accordingly. The way which I used was according to what I have already declared : *Viz.* By Diet-drinks, Baths, ointments, and herbs to wear about her neck, as is before expressed. All the herbs used were Solary and gathered at the true planetary hour, agreeing with the number attributed to the Sun.

Note, That when the *Sun* or any other planet, whose herbs you intend to use be strong in the heavens, the lesser numbers will serve, but when they are weak then the greater numbers must be used : A planet is said to be strong when he is in essential dignities, and weak when out of dignities in the heavens, the reasons I have shown elsewhere in this Book.

Another kind of Evil, commonly called Atake.

MOst People call this kind of Evil *Atake* ; by reason, that the Patient is on the sudden perplexed with great pain, whereas usually natural infirmities first mind the Patient, before it increases to extremity, according as the influence of the afflicting Planets draws to partile aspect of the significator of the Patient ; and if a figure be set for the time, when the pain first assaults the patient, one may by the rules of Astrology easily discover from what cause the grief came, and whether natural or from Witchcraft.

The way which the Witches usually take for to afflict Man or Beast in this kind, is as I conceive, done by image or model made in the likeness of that Man or Beast they intend to work mischief upon, and by the subtlety of the Devil made at such hours and times, when it shall work most powerfully upon them by thorn, pin, or needle pricked into that Limb or part of the Image, which answers to that limb or member of the body afflicted. For *Example*, I shall relate what happened lately as I am credibly informed. An Old woman, who lived near the *Devizes* in *Wiltshire*, (she was imprisoned about the time, when I began to write this book, in *Anno* 1667 for the fact) being in a lone place was observed to stoop and employ herself in digging or making a hole in the earth. Now immediately after she was gone, they went to the place, and there found an image like a man with a thorn pricked into it, at which time there was a man in the Parish who was in great tormenting pain in one of his limbs, which by compare did answer to that limb pricked with a thorn into the image, and when they took forth the thorn, the man had present ease, but when they put the thorn in again the man was tormented. When witchcraft is wrought only by image pricked as aforesaid, the Patient is usually pained outwardly, in one limb, member, or part of the body and the swelling if any is usually white : There is no pain whatsoever more tormenting, than it, and commonly such pains are white swellings ; and usually with most people called evils or *Takes*, not thinking from what cause it comes. Yet I am of opinion and find by experience, that all white swellings are not such evils, which comes from evil persons, for it may proceed from some extraordinary distemper of the nerves, such as is the evil commonly called the Kings evil, as I have already declared. It's observable that in all kinds of evil, the more they are tampered with the worse they are ; for except the right way of remedies be applied, the Patient will be but the more tormented : I know many have lost their limbs and sometimes life, and all in regard those who have undertaken to cure them, being unskilled in the way of Astrology could not effect the cure. I have cured many, who have been taken in this condition, and to my knowledge have never failed, where the Patient was curable but when the bones, sinews, nerves, and arteries, and flesh is perished before one begins, and joints dislocated, then there can be no perfect cure expected, although some good may be wrought in staying further proceedings. There is no grief or infirmity whatsoever, but may through Witchcraft and Sorcery, by the help of the Devil be wrought upon the bodies of men and beast, and I could instance many, which I have cured. I shall mention two examples : The first being a cure done upon a Maid living at *Newton* near *Newbery* in the County of *Berks*, she lay two years bedridden, and could wag neither hand nor foot ; her father told me he had tried many Doctors, which cost him above a hundred pounds, but she was never the better, but rather the worse ; she took no sustenance, save only verjuice posset. For if at any time she took ought else, she soon did vomit it up all, her body and limbs outward, were taken in the nature of a dead Palsy and her inward parts with a great stop at the breast and stomach, her Father told me the time when she first took her bed, by which I erected a Scheme, and according to the rules of Astrology, I told her Father, I found she was taken either by Witchcraft or Sorcery, if not both, and that was the reason why the drug Doctors could not help her ; I undertook the cure at a price, and within eight weeks, I recovered both her body and limbs, and she has continued well ever since, it being above nine years ago, since the cure was done. *The Way how to cure either Witchcraft or Sorcery is set down in another place in this Book.*

The Cure was effected.

In the first place I endeavoured to *afflict the Witch* ; and then by diet drinks and ointments made of planetary herbs *antipathetical* to the afflicting planet (being *Saturn*) gathered at the planetary hours, their qualities, virtues, and numbers, corresponding ; the herbs used were under the dominion of the *Sun* and *Jupiter*. It appeared that both Witchcraft and Sorcery had been wrought upon the Maid, by reason that both her limbs outward, and body inward, were afflicted as aforesaid. *Objection*, if Witchcraft works alone only but upon one limb or member of the body as before is declared ; then how comes it to pass, that her whole body and limbs generally were thus made useless, To which I answer that if the thorn, pin or needle were pricked in the head, when the sign that is the *Moon* was in *Aries* and that the infortunes as instance *Saturn* were in bad aspect to her (as probably it was) when the Witch first began her mischief, then it might unhappily work mischief or damage to the whole body : for it stands by good reason that if the brain, which is the fountain from whence the Nerves proceed be oppressed, that then the motion of the whole body must needs be obstructed, for the Nerves which is a small string that runs under the veins throughout the whole frame of the body proceeding from the brain are the only sensitive part of motion ; insomuch that if a Surgeon happen to prick a nerve, when he lets any one blood, the limb will be in danger to be useless, and I heard of two, who lost the use of their arms thereby. When I lived in *Oxford*, and as it fared with the body to be senseless and so useless, when the brain and nerves are oppressed, so likewise it fared with the body, as being dead, and void of life, when the heart and arteries are oppressed. I shall instance one example hereof, about eight or nine years ago I cured a Maid, whose name was *Mary Boyer*, she was about eighteen years of age, her Father, together with this maid lived in *Glassenbury*, being above eight miles from my dwelling : he brought her to my house where I now dwell to be cured ; her condition was as follows, Every day near the same hour she was taken with a great pain and pricking at her heart, and then immediately, sounding fits followed, lasting two or three hours ; she was above twelve months in this condition before I undertook the cure ; and as her Father told me, he had been at great charge going after many Doctors, and yet notwithstanding, was rather worse, than any whit amended, and no marvel, for how can any Doctor cure such distempers, when they are ignorant of the cause, for Witchcraft or Sorcery can no way be discovered, nor yet cured, but by the way of *Astrology*, except a Miracle be wrought, 'tis true, God can do what he pleases ; but I never knew, or heard of any Man or Beast that was cured (since the

Apostles times) that were bewitched, any other way, than by the *Astrological* way of Physick : and 'tis a great mercy, that God is pleased to raise up, and to give knowledge to a mortal man to do it ; for, although the afflictions of this kind come from the Devil and his instruments, which we commonly call evils or takes, yet the cure comes by, and through Gods Blessing upon the honest industry of the *Astrologers* and *Philosophers*, who are the men only acquainted with these kinds of cures : and as it pleases God to suffer the Devil and his Instruments the Witches to afflict his people, by reason of their neglect of duty and Prayer : so again, it pleases God through Prayers joined with lawful means, to take off their power, and to return the evil back from whence it came, and so to have their infirmities and diseases cured : these cures are not done as many foolishly imagine, by such who are called white Witches, for the white Witches and the black Witches are all one, as I shall make appear, and 'tis but a mere cheat or delusion, for the one Witch by image or model afflicts the Patient by thorn, pin, or needle pricked into it. The other Witch being Confederate gives forth, that she can cure, whereupon, when the Patient comes, these two confederate Witches divides the gain, and the cure is quickly done, for 'tis but pulling forth the thorn or pin, out of the image, and the Patient is cured ; but I have known sometimes when the Patients have been ill of long Continuance and so the grief being gotten into the flesh, bones, blood, nerves, arteries and the like, that then they could not cure them, for then Remedies proper made with planetary herbs, as diet-drinks, baths, ointments, and such like remedies, as I have elsewhere expressed, must be used, for 'tis not enough when gotten into the flesh and blood, to take out the thorn or pin ; and those who go to such cunning women, if they stay too long as aforesaid, are afterwards enforced to come to me, or some others, who are skilled in the Art of *Astrology* and *Philosophy* for cure, for Witches cannot help them ; and I have known sometimes, that suspected Witches when they could not help their Patients have come to me for remedies, and I have cured them.

I shall relate the manner how the Cure was effected upon the Maid before mentioned, with some passages which happened thereupon.

IN the first place, for the encouragement of all such who are conversant in daily Prayer to God, I shall relate what I have proved by many examples, for in all my Practice, I could never find, that ever any man, or woman that did daily pray, especially in the morning, were ever taken in the snare of Witchcraft that day : and this maid now in question, was as a man may say, taken napping ; I shall relate the manner how she became ensnared : but first I shall declare, what happened between her father, and myself concerning her devotion : after her father and myself were agreed about the Cure, I told him, 'twas pity that she did neglect her duty towards God, for if she had used daily Prayer, she had never been brought into this condition ; he answered, that to his knowledge that could not be the cause, for she did usually every morning pray, before she went forth of her Chamber : then I told him that if she would affirm it upon oath if called thereunto, I would cure her for nothing, more especially, if she prayed that day she was took in this condition, whereupon he called in the maid and after some exhortations given, I asked her the question, she answered, that she did not pray that morning when she was taken in this condition and desired her father not to be angry and she would declare the reason of her neglect, which was as follows, her Mother being minded to brew, called her up very early in the morning to fetch water from the Conduit, now the custom is, first come, first served ; it so fell out, that this maid and another maid meeting at the place, fell together by the ears concerning who should be first served, whereupon, the other maid being worsted vowed revenge ; and the same day immediately after, she was taken in this condition, as I shall relate : now her Father told me, that the other maid lived with one who was much suspected to be a Witch, and according to my Figure which was set for the day and hour when she was first taken in this condition, I found, that she was afflicted by the Planet *Saturn*, Lord of the twelfth, which is the house of Witchcraft, which Planet, according to the rules of *Astrology* did exactly personate the suspected Witch. The power of Witchcraft was so strongly wrought upon this maid, that for twelve months together she could not go into any bed until after midnight ; besides her daily fits, which usually took her near one hour of the day as follows ; first, when the fit began it would prick about her heart, as if needles were thrust into her, and then immediately after it would disperse throughout her whole body by the arteries, and then for some hours she would seem dead : and further, the power of Witchcraft was so strong upon her, that if at any time of the day, or night, (before midnight) she did but touch any bed, she would immediately fall into a fit, as I at her first coming did make several trials. I conceive, that the Witch did not only work by Witchcraft alone, by Image pricked into the heart which by sympathy, through the subtlety of the Devil worked upon the heart and arteries of the maid, but also did use some way of Sorcery, whereby to afflict her inward parts, for she was much troubled with griping pains in her belly and stomach, whereas formerly she was healthful : now the way used for the curing of this maid, was as follows, first, according to the rules hereafter mentioned, I endeavoured to afflict the Witch to the end, she might forbear to act any further in her villainy. Secondly I made her diet drinks, by decoctions with such herbs being gathered at their right planetary hours, which were under the dominion of the *Sun* and *Jupiter*, being antipathetical to the afflicting Planet

Saturn; and likewise with those herbs I made ointments proper to comfort the heart and arteries, with cataplasms to the hand-wrists, sometimes when I found the veins high, I let her blood, fearing the arteries might be oppressed thereby, for as I have already declared the arteries and nerves run both under the veins : I likewise for a time accustomed her to eat hearts oiled, baked, or stewed, which might by sympathy help to fortify her heart : I also gave her water-gruel made with such herbs which were agreeable to her condition ; to be taken an hour after she had taken her diet-drink every morning as indeed we usually do in all distempers, according to which rules before going this maid was well and perfectly cured within ten weeks, notwithstanding, she was above twelve months in this condition before she came to me : and notwithstanding, her Father as he told me had tried many Doctors to his great charge, for as in this, so in all other kinds of evils, the more they are tampered with the worse the patient will be, except they had the knowledge by the rules of *Astrology* and *Philosophy* to understand the way of Cure.

Another kind of Evil which comes from Sorcery.

I find by experience, that there is another kind of Evil wherewith many are infected, and I shall instance one example. A woman living at a place called *Nutbeam* within mile of *Way-bill* where once a year the great fair is kept, was taken with this kind of evil as follows : the cause of this woman's distemper was from Sorcery, at by my Figure was discovered, and the party suspected was the Minister of the Parish, by my Figure described to be a man of *Saturn*, in the times of *Mercury*, which signifies a man of reasonable stature swarthy complexion, and of a lumpish countenance, and sad or black hair ; he was a man of small wealth, only hired to execute the office or Function, for the time being : the occasion which moved him to do it, was, as the woman told me, because she would not trust him for malt; whereupon he threatened revenge, and at a gossiping feast he had the opportunity to do it, as follows ; First, he moved to have a health go round the table, and so did undertake to spice everyone's cup, but when it came to this woman's turn to drink, she observed, that he took spice out of another paper which he had prepared, pretending that it was all one : this woman told me she was not willing to take it, fearing least he should do her some mischief ; but being unwilling to disturb the company, well-hoping that his malice would not have lasted so long, she drank it, after which, before the day was ended, she began to be very ill, being taken with a great pain and gripping in her belly, and likewise every day increased in bigness of body, being grown so big as three ordinary women, insomuch, at length a reasonable horse could not well carry her. She tried many Doctors, and spent much money, but could find no help, at length hearing of me, her husband brought her to me ; she was above two years in this condition before I undertook the cure, yet notwithstanding I recovered her in about three months time, staying not only her griping pains in her belly, but also, did very much lesson the extreme growth of her body : The way which I used for her recovery was, by decoctions, ointments, baths, sweats and glisters : She was taken under *Saturn* who was Lord of the twelfth house, and in the ascendant : the cure was performed by antipathy, *viz*. with herbs under the *Sun*, *Mars*, and *Jupiter* : what herbs are good for Dropsical humours under the Planets before mentioned, you may find in this Book ; and likewise, how to make decoctions, bathes, oils, and glisters, suitable to her condition. Now concerning this Minister, I shall relate what followed, I having by my Art made some discovery, and this woman for the reasons aforesaid, justly suspecting him, both she and her husband were minded to have him before a Justice, but that I somewhat disheartened them, and told them, that the discovery which I had made, could be no evidence against him, whereby to implead : but not long after, this Priest having upon some other occasion differed with another of his Parishioners, after Prayers ended, his Son standing in the Church-yard, this Minister came to him, took off his hat and gave him a tap on the head, saying, (before some of the Neighbours) *Thou shalt lie by it some time for thy Fathers sake* : immediately after, this Boy, being very sick, took his bed, and came no more abroad in a long time : whereupon, this Woman's Husband, and the Boy's Father resolved to prosecute against him, and accordingly, sent for a Warrant, intending to have him before a Justice, but the Priest having some notice thereof fled, and as I am informed, was never heard of to this day.

Another Cure done upon a Boy living at Throxford, in the County of Berks, who was suddenly struck dumb, and so continued during the space of three years.

I Shall in the first place relate the manner how this Boy was taken in this condition : as follows, This Boy living with his Uncle (his Father being dead) was employed to drive, and fetch home milch beasts, being kept for a dairy ; now in a morning being holy day having on his best array, being somewhat pleasant, meets with a woman, who was very much suspected to be a Witch, and minding to make sport with her, calls her old witch, demanding whether she was going, she not answering, he threw several stones at her, with that she began to be angry, and says to him (as the boy after he could speak related) sirrah I will make you hold your tongue, using many threatening speeches ; and endeavoured to run after the boy, who was too nimble on foot for her : After which time during three years, as abovesaid, he became speechless and seeming simple and so might without question have continued to this day (without miracle) had not the Astrological way been used both for the discovery and recovery of his distemper. The Friends of this boy told me they had spent much money about his cure, but to no purpose, having as they said tried many Doctors and others, insomuch that they thought him incurable : But by accident hearing of me and of the many cures by me done, the friends of this boy came to me, desiring to know whether I would undertake to help him to his speech again : I asked them if they could tell the time, when he first lost his speech, which they readily told me. It being done upon a holy day, they could the better do it, whereupon having erected a figure, according to the day or time given, I quickly found the cause of his distemper (without which there could be no cure wrought) and told them, that I was confident through Gods blessing, that I could help them. The Planet afflicting was ♄ a cold, dry, melancholy, earthy, evil Planet : the defect lay wholly in the *Uvula* or *Gargareon* ; and as men who are taken with extreme cold, which usually settles in this part, are seemingly speechless, or at least speak with little or low voice, so this boy being more vehemently afflicted under so sad a cold planet, could not speak at all : And likewise he seemed to be foolish, for there was a great cold defect in the brain and head, so well as in the *Uvula*. Now having by the Rules of Art discovered the cause so well as the distemper itself; the friends of this boy and myself agreed upon a price for the cure, which I performed in less than a month's space. The cure was effected as follows, having in the first place by the rules hereafter mentioned, endeavoured to afflict the Witch, that so she might be discouraged to act any further in her mischief. I used herbs antipathetical to the afflicting planet being *Saturn*, *viz*. Herbs under the dominion of the *Sun* and *Jupiter*, according to their numbers and virtues, being gathered at their right planetary hours, three of which herbs being under the domain of the *Sun* I caused him to wear about his neck, it being in virtue answerable to gold, and a number which properly belonged to the *Sun*, as I have shown elsewhere, and as gold is a metal under the dominion of the Sun, and has a virtue to withstand all kinds of evils, and to comfort the heart, arteries, and vital spirits, so likewise have these herbs under his dominion the like properties, as also the ruby amongst stones ; Generally all those pains, aches, distempers or afflictions, which are caused by Witchcraft are called Evils, and sometimes these kinds of Evils will turn into white kernels, swellings, proceeding from some extraordinary distempers in the nerves (as I have elsewhere expressed, and then it's usually called *the Kings Evil.*) Having collected my herbs together according to their numbers and virtues, being under the dominion of the *Sun* and *Jupiter,* as aforesaid, and caused a mixture, then out of these herbs, we usually make diet drinks, ointments, and suffumigations ; of the diet drink, I gave him three times a day, *viz.* Morning, afternoon, and night, also every morning we usually give them water-gruel made with some of those herbs about an hour after they have taken the diet drink, by which means through Gods blessing the boy within a month was cured, and has so continued ever since. I believe it will be a warning to him, how to meddle with such Creatures in a morning without prayer. I shall relate one passage, which happened between the Boy's Uncle and myself, as follows : The month being expired, which was the time set for the Boy's cure, he came to see whether the Boy could speak or no, whereupon I called in the boy and bade him speak to his uncle, which he did, desiring to know how all his friends did ; whereupon his Uncle seemed to be much troubled, and sad, for as he told me afterwards, he did verily believe, that I had infused a spirit into the boy to make him speak ; and his reason was because the Doctors and others, who had undertaken to help him (but could not) said he would never be cured, as they verily believed by any man whatsoever : whereupon the boy's Uncle desired me to keep him somewhat longer, and then he would come and bring money for the cure : The reason why he brought no money with him, was, because he did not believe I could help him ; and he made his bargain so, that if I did not cure the boy, I was to have naught for my charge and pains. And about a week after he came privately to my Servants, desiring to speak with the boy, which he did, and then, but not before he was satisfied, for the boy could both pray and readily give answers to questions. After which, about a week following, he came again with one of his Neighbours, who both heard the boy speak and pray again, and was fully satisfied, paying me, what we had agreed upon for the cure. It seems they were not only disheartened by Physicians, but also hearing that I did many times set figures, concerning Nativities, thefts, strays, and fugitives, &c. As though I had wrought the cure by unlawful means. But before we parted, I gave them both such ample satisfaction, that they went away well contented and satisfied, being joyful, that it was their good chance to come to me.

Now whether this Boy was by this woman bewitched or whether it pleased God to lay such an affliction upon the Boy. It may be a question worthy of answer ; to which I shall briefly reply in point of art, That in regard the only afflicting planet was Lord of the twelfth and an evil planet, I concluded that the infirmity might proceed from fascination or witchcraft, but not without Gods permission, for (as I have elsewhere declared) if we neglect daily prayers, we lie liable to the assaults of *Satan*, and his Instruments for the time being ; especially in our bodies : For our Saviour *Jesus Christ* taught us to pray daily, not only for bread but also to deliver us from evil, wherein, if we fail, the fault is ours.

How to make the Sympathetical Powder with the way to apply the same, for the curing of wounds, and sundry distempers: Especially such which any way concern the blood or vital spirits.

TAke of *Roman vitriol* six or eight ounces, beat it very small in a mortar, then sieve it through a fine sieve, do it when the *Sun* enters *Leo*, which is about the twelfth of *July*, then spread it finely upon an earthen glazed pan, set it daily in the heat of the *Sun* during forty days, and keep it warm at night, and be careful it takes no wet or cold, afterwards you must continually keep it dry, with this powder alone kept dry and warm, great cures may be done. I shall instance one Example, A Brother of mine living in *Southcote* near *Reading* in the time of the late war had a Mastiff Dog shot into the neck and head, with a brace of bullets. The dog being very much swelled, lay pining away and was in appearance near to death. A Gent. who came by accident having some of this powder in his pocket was desirous to make some trial thereof upon this Dog, whereupon with a linen cloth we took some of the corruption, which was about his neck, and immediately applied a small quantity of the powder to it keeping it very warm, whereupon presently the Dog revived, stood up and wagged his tail ; then presently for further trial, we laid the powder with the corruption to the air, and then the Dog fell down as dead again, shivering, and then immediately we closed it up again, and ever afterwards kept it warm, and the Dog in a short time recovered.

The Way to apply this Powder for the curing of distempers and infirmities; especially such, wherein the Blood and vital Spirits are concerned.

WHen you are minded to cure any disease or infirmity, you must by the help of this Book take notice what herbs are good to be used to cure the grief or infirmity, out of which you must take a select number according to their elemental qualities and virtues, being rightly appropriated to their several planets, and gathered at the right planetary hours, which this Book will sufficiently instruct you, dry them so that you may pound them and sieve them into fine powder. Then take the quantity of half a dram thereof, and the like quantity of the Sympathetical powder, and mix them well together in a Mortar, ever after keeping the powder warm and dry : and when you are minded to cure thereby you must warm the powder very well over a few coals, and while its warm put a small quantity of the Patient's blood into it, and mix it very well together, always keeping it warm, and so make it up in a little bag, and let the Patient wear it next their skin, that so it may always be kept warm. I have by virtue of this powder done many very great cures, and should have still continued in this way of practice, but that I found many were unsatisfied, concerning the legality thereof, taking it for a kind of charm, by reason I ordered the patient to wear it about their necks, and I believe they did the rather concept so in regard, I did use to resolve many questions in Astrology, as Thefts, Strays, Fugitives, &c. There is but one danger in this way of cure, which is as follows. If the Patient happen to lose this mixture from their necks or body wheresoever worn, or otherwise let it take cold, the grief will be apt to return again, more especially if the Patient be not perfectly recovered. But when the Patient is through well, then they may burn it. I could have inserted many cures, which I have effected by virtue of this powder, I shall only mention one for example, as follows, about nine years ago, there lived a woman in *Newbery*, in the County of *Berks*, she was daily troubled with fits, which at the first, would begin with a kind of trembling about the heart, and from thence by degrees set at the arteries to work throughout her whole body, after which, for some hours she would be as seemingly dead, and could wag neither arm or leg ; for cure whereof, I let her blood in the heart vein, and having my powders made in readiness, according to what is before expressed ; I mixed some of her blood with the powder, and while it was warm made it up into a little bag, which I caused her to wear about her neck, by virtue of which, not omitting diet-drink suitable to her condition ; she was in about a month's space recovered ; notwithstanding, she was near twelve months in this condition before she came to me : The cure being perfected, her husband, according to our agreement paid me for the cure, but it so chanced, that within some small time after, she carelessly lost this from her neck, whereupon, her fits began to mind her again, and more and more increased, insomuch, that she was almost so bad as at the first, for as I said before, except the patient be for some time perfectly well, at least a month, the grief will be apt to return, especially, when the principal matter of cure is lost or neglected, for its not sufficient in any distemper whatsoever only to cure, except for a time there be a perfect settlement, for we daily find, that relapses are very dangerous and apt to befall many who think themselves well recovered. This woman's husband came to me again, and told me, that his Wife was so bad as ever (being much discontented) he not knowing the reason ; I asked him, whether she had not lost the little bag from her neck which I gave her to wear. He told me he thought she had : the truth is, through carelessness she had lost it, whereupon, I once more let her blood, and did as is before expressed, desiring her to take care of it, which she did ; after which, she became well again, and her fits left her, and so has continued well ever since, as I am informed. This cure being effected about eight or nine years ago.

The Unguent, or wonderful Ointment for Wounds: Composed of the four Elemental parts of Man's Body. The Seven Planets being applied thereunto : Its making, and use ; follows :

The Ingredients.

The Moss of a dead Mans Skull	2 ounces.
Of Man's Grease	2 ounces.
Of Mummy	½ ounce.
Of Man's Blood	½ ounce.
Oil of Lindseed	2 ounces.
Oil of Roses	2 ounces.
Bole Armeniac	½ ounce.

The three last ingredients are the rather added to it because it helps to bring it to a subtle ointment : and without question, there is also great virtue in them.

Elements.	Nature.	Complexion.	Planets.
Water.	Cold and Moist.	Flegm.	Venus and Luna.
Fire.	Hot and Dry.	Choler.	Sol and Mars.
Earth.	Cold and Dry.	Melancholy.	Saturn & Mercury
Air.	Hot and Moist.	Sanguine.	Jupiter.

ALL these things before mentioned must be mixed together and beaten well in a mortar until it become an ointment then keep it in a close thing from air for your use. The way to use this Unguent whereby to cure, is as follows : Take the blood or matter of the Wound upon the Weapon or Instrument which made the Wound : or otherwise, dry it upon a piece of wood, then put the wood into the ointment, or else anoint the blood, being kept dry upon the wood with the ointment, and keep it from air ; you must every day wet a fresh linen rag with the Urine of the Patient, and so bind up the wound : do it early every morning. Also you must be very careful that the ointment which is applied to the blood take no cold, with this Unguent wonderful things may be done if it be rightly managed according to the directions aforesaid. I shall quote one example concerning the trial of this Unguent as follows, One day being at dinner with Sir *Humphrey Forrester* of *Aldermaston* in the County of *Berks*. The Gentlewoman, who usually waited on his Lady was extremely tormented with the toothache, we caused her to prick her tooth with a toothpick, and to bleed it, immediately we put the toothpick into the ointment, and the Gentlewoman had present ease ; after some short time, we took forth the toothpick, and put it into vinegar, whereupon she was presently in extreme pain : We took the toothpick forth of the vinegar, and applied it to the unguent, and she was immediately well, and so continued. I could have inserted many great cures done by virtue of this unguent, which for brevity's sake only I am willing to omit.

Concerning Witchcraft, and Sorcery, with the cure thereof, as follows.

THe way to know whether the patient be bewitched or not I have already set down, elsewhere in this Book. I find by experience, that those who are taken in the snare of witchcraft are usually afflicted in some outward limb or member of the body caused by an image made in the likeness of man or beast, and through the subtlety of the Devil made at such hours and times, when by sympathy it shall reflect upon the man or beast whom they intend to hurt or destroy ; it being done by thorn, pin, or needle pricked into that part of the image, which answers to that part of the body of man or beast wherein they are pained or grieved. An *Example* hereof I have already mentioned, concerning the Woman lately taken at the *Deviszes* in *Wiltshire* : But that which I conceive is the most usual way practised by Witches is most properly called Sorcery : For by the help of the Devil some poisonous matter is prepared, and mixed with some blood and vital spirit of the Witch, and so by smell or taste infused into the body of man or beast bewitched, or rather by which they are infected : For it's observable in Philosophy : *Si acceperis terram candaverosam cujuseunque viri mulierisve, qui notabili quocunque morbo moriebatur, eandemque des ullo masculo aut foeminae, eodem morbo contaminabuntur ; in morbis aliqusbus odore tantum hoc efficitur, Exempla gratia, in peste, Lue Venerea, seu morbi Gallico Elephantiasi sive Lepra.**

Those who are thus wrought upon by sorcery may be infected with most kinds of diseases whatsoever : As I have sufficiently discovered in my *Practice of Physick*. Besides I have known many things, which through sorcery have been so infected and spoiled, as instance bear cream, and milk, whey, and such like, that neither Housewife or Dairy Maid could make any good use thereof. I shall relate one *Example* hereof when I was a Boy my Father kept a Dairy at a place called *Shenfield* near *Reading*, and one of my Sisters had the charge thereof, upon a time my Father desired her to make some wild curds, and to send them home ; which she endeavoured to do, but could make none. The reason was, as she conceived because an Old woman (suspected for a Witch) was at that

---

*Translation: *If you should ingest the dirt of a corpse, male or female, which died of a disease, you can infect others, even if they only smelled your odor. For example, the plague, syphilis or leprosy can be transmitted by this means.* (Thanks to Philip Graves.) Why the author thought this worthy of Latin is unclear. Perhaps he means to say that not all those accused of witchcraft were actually guilty, that some, perhaps, were unwitting "Typhoid Marys". — *Editor*

time denied whey, who went muttering away discontented. The next day my Father came with one of his Brothers, named *John Blagrave*, a man of great knowledge in Astrology and Philosophy, as appears by his many works in print. Now my Father asked her why she sent him no curds, she told him, she could make none, notwithstanding she had used her best skill ; and related what is aforesaid concerning the Woman suspected : Now my Father's Brother aforesaid being desirous to make further trial hereof went into the House, and caused the whey to be hung over the fire again which no sooner was done, but presently it rumbled, and made a noise, as if many bullets had been in it, whereupon he caused the Kettle and whey to be taken from the fire, and caused a greater fire to be made : He also called for a cord and an iron wedge, he took the cord, and bound the Kettle round about, and wrestled it very hard, and then caused the Kettle with whey to be set over the fire again, and having heated the wedge red hot, put him into the whey, and immediately there was abundance of curds rose up, after which my Uncle sent a messenger to the suspected Witch's house to know how she did, who brought word, that after much knocking at length she opened the door, where he found the Witch or suspected person shrunk up like a purse or leather put into the fire. By which it appeared, that part of the vital spirit of the Witch was infused into the whey, for otherwise it could not have wrought so violently upon her, for should the poisonous matter, or thing be given or used alone without some blood or vital spirit of the Witch mingled with it, the burning of the patients blood or urine would not hurt them, or the putting this red hot wedge into the whey, could no way have afflicted her, which it did by Sympathy ; as appeared by her body being shrunk up as aforesaid.

The true way to Cure both Witchcraft and Sorcery, according to the Author's experience and Practice.

THe curing of such who are bewitched, is not done only by such, who are called white Witches (as many foolish do imagine) for the white Witch and the black Witch are all one, as I have elsewhere expressed, they are but confederate Witches, the one Witch by thorn, pin, or needle pricks into the Image through the subtlety of the Devil causing the infirmity, pain, or lameness ; the other Witch gives forth, that she can cure, and so when the friends of the bewitched comes to the white Witch, or cunning woman (they divide the gain) and the cure is quickly done, it's but pulling forth, the thorn, pin or needle, and the Patient is cured, and I have been credibly informed by some who have gone to these cunning women, or white Witches ; that their Cattle, or the Patient afflicted have been perfectly well before they have gotten home : but as I have already declared, after either man or beast have been bewitched above month, they cannot cure them, especially, if the pain continue in one place all that time but sometimes they will move the thorn, pin, or needle into some other part of the body, that so they may have remedy when they come to them ; for after the pain or infirmity have been of above a month standing, the grief will get into the flesh, blood and vital parts, and then the pulling forth of the thorn, and the rest will do the Patient but little good, and cannot possibly help them, wherefore in this condition the Patients friends must of necessity repair to such who are well skilled in *Astrological* and *Philosophical* way of cure as I shall declare in order hereunto, but before we proceed to the way of cure, it will be necessary to show, how to afflict the Witch, that so she may be discouraged to act any further in her mischief : for notwithstanding their witchcraft by image, as aforesaid, yet I seldom find, especially where the Patient has been above a month bewitched, but that Sorcery is wrought so as witchcraft, upon the Patient ; and sometimes immediately together with the Witchcraft, especially, where there are no confederate Witches, for the white Witches cannot help, where Sorcery has been wrought upon the Patient, by reason it breaks forth immediately into some Poisonous or infectious inward grief or infirmity, which can no way be cured (except by accident) but by the *Astrological, Philosophical* way of Physick.

Here follows some experimental Rules, whereby to afflict the Witch, causing the evil to return back upon them.

1. ONe way is by watching the suspected party when they go into their house ; And then presently to take some of her thatch from over the door, or a tile, if the House be tiled ; if it be thatch you must wet and sprinkle it over with the patient's water, and likewise with white salt, then let it burn or smoke through a trivet, or the frame of a skillet : you must bury the ashes that way, which the suspected Witch lives. It's best done either at the change, full, or quarters of the *Moon* : Or otherwise, when the Witch's significator is in *Square* or *Opposition* to the *Moon*. But if the Witch's house be tiled, then take a tile from over the door, heat him red hot, put salt into the patient's water, and dash it upon the red hot tile, until it be consumed, and let it smoke through a trivet or frame of a skillet, as aforesaid.

2. Another way is to get two new horseshoes, heat one of them red hot, and quench him in the patients urine, then immediately nail him on the inside of the threshold of the door with three nails, the heel being upwards : then having the patient's urine set it over the fire, and set a trivet over it, put into it three horse nails, and a little white salt : Then heat the other horseshoe red hot, and quench him several times in

the urine, and so let it boil and waste until all be consumed; do this three times and let it be near the change, full, or quarters of the Moon; or let the Moon be in *Square* or *Opposition* to the Witch's Significator.

3. Another way is to stop the urine of the Patient, close up in a bottle, and put into it three nails, pins, or needles, with a little white Salt, keeping the urine always warm: If you let it remain long in the bottle, it will endanger the witch's life: for I have found by experience, that they will be grievously tormented making their water with great difficulty, if any at all, and the more if the *Moon* be in *Scorpio* in *Square* or *Opposition* to his Significator, when it's done.

4. Another way is either at the new, full, or quarters of the moon; but more especially, when the *Moon* is in *Square* or *Opposition* to the Planet, which personates the Witch, to let the patient blood, and while the blood is warm, put a little white salt into it, then let it burn and smoke through a trivet. I conceive this way does more afflict the Witch, than any of the other three beforementioned by reason the blood has more life in it than the urine; for the urine is accounted, but as the excrement of blood: The reason why the Witch is tormented, when the blood or urine of the patient is burned, is because there is part of the vital spirit of the Witch in it, for such is the subtlety of the Devil, that he will not suffer the Witch to infuse any poisonous matter into the body of man or beast, without some of the Witches blood mingled with it, as appears by the whey before mentioned. For 'tis the Devil's policy, either by this means to detect them or otherwise by torment to bring them to their ends: for the devil well knows, that when the blood or urine of the patient is burned, that the Witch will be afflicted, and then they will desire to come to the place, for to get ease, for by the smell thereof, their pain is mitigated by

sympathy ; even as by sympathy, when the blood and urine is burning, they are tormented, yet sometimes they will rather endure the misery of it than appear, by reason country people oft times will fall upon them, and scratch and abuse them shrewdly. I conceive the only reason the devil sucks the Witch's blood is merely to detect them, or otherwise one way or other to bring them to their ends, and sometimes they are discovered by their teat, at which place the Devil usually sucks their blood, whereby to mix with the poison, which they by their wicked ways infuse into the body of man or beast, and so infect them. I find by practice and experience that few or none are bewitched by Image or Model alone, but that there is Sorcery wrought with it for otherwise the burning of the blood or urine of the patient could no way afflict them in any sympathetic way, as aforesaid ; having by the rules aforegoing set forth the way, how to afflict the Witch. I shall in the next place discover the general way of cure.

The way to cure both Witchcraft and Sorcery, commonly called Evils or Takes.

Having by a figure discovered under what planet the Patient is afflicted, and in what part of the body the grief or pain lies ; whether outward in any limb or part of the body, or throughout the whole body, as it will sometimes fall out when the Nerves or Arteries are oppressed, proceeding from the heart and brain, or whether inward in the bowels, guts, liver, lungs, heart, breast, or stomach ; or be it what other disease or distemper whatsoever, for as I have already declared there is no disease or distemper whatsoever, but may be brought upon man or beast by witchcraft and Sorcery, as I have already in several examples demonstrated : If the grief, pain, or distemper, be in the outward parts, limbs, or members of the body, then the cure must be by baths and ointments made antipathetical to the afflicting planets ; As instance if *Saturn* be the afflicting planet, then herbs must be used under the *Sun* and *Jupiter*. If *Mars* be the afflicting planet, then herbs must be used under the dominion of the *Sun* and *Venus* : Always provided that the herbs be gathered at the right planetary hours, according to their virtues and numbers : If the grief lies inward at the breast, stomach, and heart, then you must choose such herbs, which are under the dominion of that planet, which is antipathetical to the afflicting planet, and are good to open obstructions, and to comfort the heart and arteries, ever remembering in all cures to use a select number of herbs, under the dominion of the *Sun*, in regard he governs the heart and is fountain of life, and sole Monarch of the heavens. If the grief lie in the bowels and guts, then sometimes glisters must be used made with such herbs especially which are good to expel poison, being under the dominion of *Sol*, which this book will sufficiently instruct you in, together with such herbs, which are of a contrary nature to the afflicting planet, but if the afflicting planet is more strong than the planet which is a contrary nature, then you must choose a small select number of herbs of his own nature, which are good to cure the infirmity, and mix them with the other herbs beforementioned, concerning the way to make glitters, baths, oils, decoctions, or diet drinks, and what else is meet to be used in all cures whatsoever, I have already elsewhere in this book expressed.

Note, That in the curing of all kinds of evils, I usually cause the patients to wear a select number of solary herbs gathered at the hour of the *Sun*, the reasons I have shown elsewhere in this book. I could have been more copious in setting forth the way of curing both witchcraft and sorcery, but that I have sufficiently treated thereof in the way of curing all kinds of evils beforementioned, for I conceive, that generally those evils beforementioned, came from witchcraft and Sorcery, only some particular evils may proceed from some extraordinary distemper of the nerves as I have elsewhere expressed with the reasons thereof.

Here follows some notable Philosophical Secrets worthy our knowledge.

How by the Magnet of one's Body to extract a Spiritual Mummy whereby to cure most Diseases incident to the body of Man : It being done either by semination or transplantation hereof into a growing vegetable, as follows.

THe *Magnet* of one's body is the Dung or Excrement, which must be dried seven or nine days in the shade, and kept from wet. This *Magnet* thus prepared must be laid to that part of the body which naturally evacuates by sweat from the vital or natural part of the body defective. But if we make a general medicine, then the *Magnet* may be applied to all parts, which naturally evacuate by sweat. This *Magnet* must be so prepared, that we may transplant the same, when the *Moon* increases, and if she apply from that planet, which is Lord of the Ascendant of the patient, or from the planet afflicting to one of the fortunes, 'twil work the stronger, provided that the fortune, which the *Moon* applies to be *antipathetical* to the afflicting planet ; as if *Mars* be the afflicting planet then let the *Moon* apply to *Venus*, if *Saturn* afflicts then to *Jupiter*, if the Lord of the ascendant or the afflicting planet be a fortune, then let the *Moon* apply to the other fortune, the manner how to transplant the imbibed *Magnet* whereby to cure by semination is, as follows : Take the imbibed *Magnet*, and mix it with a reasonable quantity of earth, and then sow in it such seeds of herbs which are proper to cure the infirmity, which this book will sufficiently instruct you in. Let the earth thus mingled be placed in as fruitful a place as conveniently you can, that it may grow the better, you must sometimes more especially, when the *Moon* is in *Conjunction, Trine,* or *Sextile* of the *Sun* or one of the fortunes, mix the patient's water with some of their excrements and so water the seeds, but you must not do it too often, once a week will be enough, for fear you should destroy the seed, for the rain and other fertile waters will be most proper and natural to make it grow.

There is yet another way, by me used, which is to take the imbibed earth, prepared as aforesaid : And having a plant, which either by sympathy or antipathy is most rational to cure the infirmity taken up clean with its root, place it into the imbibed earth, and so water it as aforesaid : Both ways are effectual to cure if rightly ordered. Lastly, when you find that by semination, or transplantation, the grief is changed into a vegetable, we must do as follows ; If the disease be dry, and of a combust nature, as the yellow jaundies or the like ; then you must take the herbs or plants with its earth and cast them into running water : If the disease be of moisture, then burn the earth and plants. If the grief be airy, then hang the earth and plants in the smoke to dry, and the Patient will be firmly cured.

How to Care any Swelling, Sore, Schirrous Tumor, or Warts.

TAke the flesh, hand, or any part of any man that is newly dead, with it rub or stroke any place defective, and then bury it : As the dead man's hand or flesh perishes or wastes in the earth, so the swelling, sore, or schirrous tumor, or warts will fade away, and the Patient be recovered. The reason in Philosophy is thus, as the northern property is an enemy to southern heat, so by his contact it causes all unnatural things growing to fade away, in changing the vegetating nature growing touched, into the mortifying nature dying.

How to work the same Cure by Herbs or Plants.

TAke *Arsmart* or *Adders-tongue* gather it at the hour of *Mars* the Moon increasing, let *Mars* be in *Trine* or *Sextile* to *Venus* or the Moon applying from *Mars* to *Venus*, or from *Venus* to *Mars* ; steep the herb or weed first in fair water, until it be well moistened, then apply it to the place defective, until it be warm, after which bury the plant or weed, and as it perishes in the earth, so the Patient will recover.

How to Cure an Atrophy or wasting Limb.

BOre a hole in a *Willow-tree* with an augur to the pith ; save some of the bored stuff, and apply it to the limb or Member of the body defective, at the new of the *Moon* 24 hours, then take the paring of the nails, with some hair, and the scraping of the skin from the limb or member of the body defective, put all these into the hole of the tree, and stop them up close with a peg of the same wood, do this when *Saturn* is weak, the *Moon* increasing, the fortunes in some friendly Aspect to the *Moon*, in fruitful Signs : Also a hole bored in the root of a Hazel tree, and ordered as aforesaid, the bark being taken off, and laid on again, and then covered with earth will do it.

How to cure the hot or cold Gout.

BOre a hole in an Oak to the pith, then take the bored stuff and apply it to the Limb or member defective, three days before the change of the *Moon* ; then take the pairing of the nails, and hair of the Limb or Member defective, and put it together with the bored stuff into the hole of the tree, and stop it up close with a peg of the same wood : do this, when *Saturn* is weak, if the Gout be of cold, or when *Mars* is weak if the Gout be of heat, and let the *Moon* be in *Trine* or *Sextile* to *Venus* : if the Gout be of heat, or to *Jupiter* if the Gout be of cold, you must be lure to stop it up close, and semon [seal?] it up from air.

How to Cure a Plague-Sore, and draw forth the venomous matter.

TAke a living Chick and apply the Fundament of the Chick to the Plague-sore, it will draw forth the Venom, kill the Chick and cure the Patient. Also a dried Toad macerated in Vinegar, and laid to the sore will draw forth the venomous matter, and cure the Patient.

How to cure the Hernia, or Rupture.

BOre a hole in an Oak to the pith : but first so, take off the bark that it may glutinate and grow : lay on the bored stuff to the place defective three days and nights before the new *Moon*; then take some hair from the privy parts, together, with the pairing of the nails, and the bored stuff, and put them into the Oak, and so stop it up with a peg of the same tree, then lay on the bark, and with tree-wax, or tempered clay, or paste, cement and daub the place up from air : And as the bark glutinates and grows, the Hernia, or Rupture will close ; also a hole bored in the root of a Hazel tree will do it, being ordered as aforesaid, and kept close covered with earth ; this is best done in the spring quarter by reason the bark will glutinate and close the better.

Here follows two pretty Secrets in Philosophy.

How to know how any kinsman, friend, or acquaintance does during their absence, being traveled into any far Country.

YOu must cause your Kinsman, or Friend to be let blood, and while its warm, infuse a small quantity of the Spirit of Wine into it, and keep it close stopped up in a glass from air ; now if your friend be well and contented, the blood will look lively and fresh accordingly, but if he chance to be ill, or discontented, the blood will be changed, and the more ill or discontented your friend is, the more will the blood be changed accordingly ; If he be much perplexed, vexed, or feverish the blood will be high coloured ; if melancholy, weak and faint, the blood will be pale and wan. And after sickness, if he recover health, the blood will look lively and fresh again, as at the first ; but if they happen to die, the blood will putrefy and stink accordingly, as will the rest of his body.

How to know each other's mind at a distance, it being done by Sympathy of motion as follows.

LEt there be two Needles made of one and the same Iron, and by one and the same hand, and touched by one and the same Loadstone. Let them be framed *North*, and *South*, when the *Moon* is in *Trine* to *Mars*, and applying to one of the fortunes : the Needles being made, place them in concave boxes, then make two Circles answerable to the Diameters of the Needles, divide them into twenty four equal parts, according to the number of letters in the Alphabet then place the letters in order round each Circle, now when you desire to make known each other's mind, the day and hour being first concluded on before hand ; you must upon a table or some convenient place fix your boxes with the Needles fixed therein, then having in readiness pen, ink, and paper, and with each party a Loadstone, those who intends first to begin, must with his Loadstone gently cause the Needle to move from one letter to another, until a word is perfected, according to which motion the other needle will answer : and then after some small stay, they must begin another word, and so forward until his mind is known. Which being done, the other friend with his Loadstone must do as before, moving gently from letter to letter until he has returned answer accordingly : this will hold true if rightly managed.

Here follows some Practical and Experimental Rules whereby to give judgment Astrologically, either upon Thefts, Strays, Fugitives, Decumbitures of sick Persons, or Urines, or any other Horary Question Whatsoever.

IN regard it has been my custom together with my daily practice in Physick for many years past, by the rules of *Astrology*, not only to give Judgment upon Decumbitures and Urines of sick persons, but also upon Nativities ; and to resolve all Horary Questions, as Thefts, Strays amongst Cattle, and Fugitives, and by reason whereof, many foolish and ignorant people, and others, who think themselves wise also have rashly and inadvisedly judged my ways and actions of this nature, to be Diabolical ; and thereupon, have not only themselves refused to come or send to me for help, in case of sickness, but have also diverted others upon the like occasions whereupon to satisfy both

Astrological judgment upon theft 151

my friends, and others, Antagonists ; I have inserted these Judgments following, according to the rules of *Astrology*, which may serve, together with other directions in this Book elsewhere expressed, if well heeded ; not only to satisfy the learned in this Art, concerning the legality of my way of Practice herein, but also to instruct others who are young students in this Art : I could have inserted Figures for every question, having many hundreds lying by me, but being unwilling to spend time, or blot paper therewith, presuming that what I have written will be sufficiently satisfactory to each friendly Reader, yet for further satisfaction I shall refer the desirous herein to my *Ephemeris* for the year, 1658, Wherein I have not only by Scripture, and reason vindicated the Art of *Astrology*, but also have inserted therein three Schemes with judgments *Astrological* thereupon, The one concerning strays amongst Cattle : The second, concerning Thefts : The third, concerning Sickness : I confess I have denied many, concerning questions of Thefts, for it neither brings credit, nor yet much gain to the Artist : for let a man be never so exact herein what will they for the most part say ? If by the Art we discover the thief, and way of the goods, surely he does it by the Devil, how could he so exactly else discover the Thief and way of the goods ; but if we chance to miss, as sometimes we may do by taking a wrong ascendant ; and more especially, when a wrong time is given for the time of loosing : then they will assuredly say : we do but cozen and cheat people of their money, besides it oft times brings trouble to the Artist : I shall relate one accident which befell me herein : Once a *Butcher* of our Parish having lost some linen, and linen Clothes, came with his wife to my house, desiring me to Erect a Figure, and thereby to inform him who had it, or what became of the linen ; Now by the Figure, I described a Maid servant who lived in the house ; when he came home, he inadvisedly called his Maid thief, saying, she had stolen his linen, whereupon, she goes to the Justice for a

Warrant, to bring her Master before him, pretending, that he had done her much wrong, in defaming her ; now, her Master to excuse himself, laid the fault on me ; whereupon, I was sent for by Warrant, to appear at a day set, which accordingly I did, where I met with a Minister of *Reading*, who was a great enemy to *Astrology*, who, as I was informed, came on purpose to aggravate the matter against me, maintaining, that the Art was Diabolical ; whereupon having heard all my accusations with many vile reproaches, with so much patience as possibly I could, I at length, desired the Justice that I might be heard, and not interrupted until he had fully heard what I could say, which was granted ; whereupon in the first place, as touching the Maid, I told the Justice that what I said to the Butcher, was no more than what I discovered by the Art of *Astrology*, which Art was known, and allowed in all Schools of learning through the World ; and that I could both by Scripture, and reason prove it to be Lawful, if I might be heard ; the Minister replied, he would maintain the contrary, I asked him, if he would argue it with me in point of Art, which I thought he understood not ; or, in Divinity, that which he professed. He said, by Divinity, I answered, that I was content : after some arguments I desired his answer, concerning the I. of *Samuel*, the 9 Chapter Where we find that *Saul, together with one of his Father's Servants was sent forth to search for his Father's Asses that was lost, who after three days search in the Wilderness could not find them : whereupon, they communed together what to do, who concluded, to go to the Seer which was Samuel the Prophet* : For Prophets, as the Marginal Notes testifies, were sometimes called *Seers* without question, a byword given them as sometimes *Astrologers* are called Cunning-men : But says *Saul* to the Servant, *What have we to give the man* ? by which it appears, they thought he would take money (and good reason for his pains) *the servant answered, I have four shekels, then come says Saul, let us go* ; and when they came to *Samuel*, after some communication, he tells than, *the*

Asses are found and at home, bidding them, return in peace. The Minister hearing this after some pause, said, *Samuel* was to blame : Now the matter of discovering goods lost was the only thing urged against me (for he could not be ignorant of the strong influence which the Stars and Planets have upon all sublunary Creatures in other regards :) The Justice hearing his weak reply, told him plainly, that for ought he could perceive, I was too hard for him, and wished him to give over his discourse, unless he could produce better matter ; not long after, notwithstanding this Maid's impudence, maintaining the contrary against her Master and Dame and myself : at a fair she was apprehended at *Reading* and brought before the same Justice with some of her Dame's linen clothes upon her, and then she kneeled down and begged for mercy, but what punishment she had, or what became of her afterwards I never inquired, neither do I desire as I said before, to be troubled with such questions.

Of Horary Questions.

BY a Horary Question, any one matter or thing may be resolved which concerns the querent, provided, that the ascendant, together with its Lord or Planet posited in the ascendant, or Sign where the Lord of the ascendant is, personates the querent : and that the figure be radical. There is no matter or thing whatsoever, but will be concerned in one of the twelve houses : as for example, if it concerns the querent's person, then the first house is it ; if his estate the second house ; if his kindred or neighbours, the third house ; if his Father, or lands, or dwellings, or the end of any thing, the fourth house ; if his children play, messengers, or agents, then the fifth house ; if his servants, sickness, or small cattle, the sixth house ; if love questions, his wife, public enemies, or thefts, the seventh house ; if wills, legacies, the dowry of the wife, or manner of death, the eighth house ; if long voyages, or journeys, church matters, religion, or dreams, the ninth house ; if honour, office, or preferment, then the tenth house ; if his friends, the eleventh house ; if private enemies, great cattle, or witches, then the twelfth house ; there may be many other matters or things resolved by the twelve houses, but these are the most usual, and material.

Of Thefts and Stray amongst Cattle.

THere are two ways in giving judgment, in case of losses : The one is by Erecting a Scheme for the time of a thing being lost or strayed, or otherwise ; if the party be present that lost the goods, or that was trusted with the goods, to take the present time when first the question was propounded, and so to Erect a Figure, taking care that it be radical, and that the ascendant together with its Lord, or Planet posited in the ascendant personates the Querent ; If it concerns Cattle or any other thing lost or missed, and that the querent is uncertain, whether it be stolen, strayed , or casually lost, you must in this case examine by an *Ephemeris*, or Almanack, which has the daily motions of the Planets , whether the Lord of the first, or second house, or Lord of part of Fortune, or the Lord of the house of the *Moon*, or of her term, separates from any Planet by any Aspect whatsoever ; then you may conclude, that the thing is not stolen : All Planets which are lowest in their Spheres, are said to separate from a higher Planet when they depart from them by any Aspect whatsoever ; But if a higher Planet happen to be Retrograde, that is, going backward in motion, then the higher Planet may be said, to separate from a lower ; Now if on the contrary you find, that neither the Lord of the Ascendant, or second house ; or Lord of part of Fortune, or Lord of the house of the *Moon* or of his term, separates from other Planets, but that other Planets separate from them, then we may conclude, that the Cattle or thing lost is stolen, if the separations be near equal, then the Plurality of testimonies must be regarded ; if you find by the rules before going, that the Cattle or thing missed, is strayed or casually lost and not stolen ; then you must have regard to the *Moon*, & Lord of the twelfth, if it be great Cattle; or to the Lord of the sixth, if it be small Cattle, as Sheep Hogs, Goats, and such like ; and observe what signs the *Moon*, and Lord of the house of the Cattle are in ; or part of fortune, or his Lord, and judge by the strongest ; and then observe the nature of the Sign, whether Fiery, Earthy, Airy, or Watery, and what places they represent and then observe, whether the Planets be in Angles, succedent or cadent houses and whether in moveable, fixed, or common Signs ; and how many Signs or Degrees there are, between the Ascendant and Planet which represents the Cattle lost and so judge accordingly ; fixed Signs, and cadent houses always signify the greatest distances, and we usually allow for every fixed Sign, four miles ; for common signs, and succedent houses we usually allow somewhat above half so much as we do for fixed signs, that is about two miles and a half for every common Sign ; moveable Signs and Angles shows the Cattle to be near the place, and for every moveable Sign we usually allow but half a mile : Now had the goods lost been Gold Rings, or Gold, Plate, or Silver, or Linen, or Precious Stones, as Rubies, or Diamonds, or the like ; then we must take notice, what Sign the Lord of the second is in, and likewise, what sign the part of Fortune is in, and his Lord ; also the Lord or significator of the thing lost, what sign he is in, as if Gold which is under the *Sun*, or Silver under the *Moon*, or Linen under *Venus*, likewise a Diamond is under *Venus* ; and the Ruby under the *Sun* ; also the fourth house, and his Lord are to be regarded, as showing the end of all things, and you must judge according to the Plurality of testimonies ; if the significators be in Fiery Signs, it shows, the goods lost to be near the Fire, or Chimney ; if in Earthy Signs, then in some low place, or with earth ; if in Watery Signs, then in, or near some Water, as sink, pump, or cistern, or such like : if in Airy Signs, then above stairs or, in some high place. But if on the contrary, by the rules aforesaid you find the thing stole, then the description of the thief, and what became of the goods, is as follows ; first the thief is described by that Planet which is peregrine in an Angle, if no peregrine Planet be in an Angle, or second house, then the Lord of the seventh house shall be significator of the thief, sometimes the Lord of the hour will do it, when the time of losing is certainly known. If many peregrine Planets be in Angles ; more especially when a double bodied Sign ascends, then it shows so many thieves. A Planet is said to be peregrine, when he is out of all essential dignities, *viz.* neither in his house, exaltation, triplicity, term, or face, having found by *Ptolemy's* Table in the Almanack what Planet or Planets are peregrine, you may describe their persons in this Book, under the title of the Bodily Shape, and which of the Planets generally rule. The way of the goods if found thus, if the Lord of the second house, and significator of the thief be joined together, or have any friendly Aspect to each other, or be in one triplicity, or if the significator of the thief disposes of the Querent's part of Fortune, or the Lord of the second house, or the significator of the goods, Then we may conclude, that the goods are with the thief, and at his disposing ; but if the significator of the Thief be separated from what is aforesaid, and applies ; or if the *Moon*, or any other inferiour planet separates from the significator of the Thief and applies to another planet, he shall be the receiver, which is signified by that planet, you must judge the way and distance of the thief according to the signs and quarters of Heaven, where the significator of the thief is accounting from the ascendant, as is before expressed.

Of Fugitives.

AS in questions of thefts and strays, so the like in Fugitives, judgement is given either by erecting a scheme, for the time of straying or going away, or otherwise, for the time of the querent's coming : If you have the exact time of the fugitive's going away. Then the Ascendant, its Lord, the Moon and Planet posited in the ascendant or angle, especially if he personate the fugitive, shall be significators of the fugitive, and according to the Nature of the Signs, and places by them signified and quarters of heaven, wheresoever we find them together with their applications to other Planets judgement is usually given : If those significators be in or apply to the sign *Gemini*, then we conclude they are travelled towards *London*, if in *Capricorn* then *Oxford* ; if in *Virgo*, *Reading* ; if *Cancer*, *Scotland* ; if *Taurus*, *Ireland* ; if the principal significator as in the ninth house, or joined to the Lord of the ninth, then we conclude they are for a voyage or long intended journey : north signs show northward, East Signs eastward, West signs westward, South signs southward : Always observing the quarter of heaven : If the planets concerned be swift in motion, and in movable signs, then they go apace, if in fixed signs and slow in motion then they go but slow ; but if the time of flying be not perfectly known, then we erect the figure according to the time when the question was propounded, and so the Lord of the seventh house joining there with *Mercury* and the *Moon*, but more especially that planet, which owns the fugitive according to shape and profession : also we must consider what relation the fugitive has to the querent, whether wife or husband, kindred or servant and the like, and if the personal shape of the fugitive corresponds with the planet which is Lord of the house inquired after, you may with the more confidence give judgement thereby. I have ofttimes given judgement upon these questions, and find they will hold true, if well heeded.

Of Urines.

THe Astrological way whereby to give judgement at the view or first sight of the urine, both in acute and chronic griefs, is immediately to erect a figure, and so to vary your Ascendant that it may be radical and that the ascendant together with its Lord may personate the sick, and if the griefs be acute, then the time of decumbiture or first falling ill, must be inquired after, that so the assured place of the *Moon* in any of the twelve Signs may be obtained, for by the *Moon* in any of the twelve Signs afflicted of the infortunes, the grief is discovered together with its cause and termination. But if the grief be chronic that is of above a Month's standing then from the *Sun* the ascendant sixth house and their Lords afflicted, judgment is usually given. In regard I have already at large set forth my way of practice herein, I shall in this place only in brief set down, what I find concerning my experience in urines, for although an exact judgement both concerning the grief, together with its cause and termination (by urine) cannot be obtained, yet some general judgements thereby may be given, which may well serve for a four penny reward : First if the urine be of an amber colour (and the patient ill) for generally that coloured urine shows health of body. Then the grief or infirmity lies in the vital and animal spirits from whence proceed palsies, palpitations, and convulsions, and such like distempers : In this condition the urine is not concerned by reason the blood and those passages from whence the urine proceeds, are not infected, for the urine is but the excrement of blood ; if the urine be white or palish, it shows great weakness both in stomach and body, and if the urine be high coloured and red, it argues a fever, or that some extraordinary pain afflicts the Sick, but the place where and cause why cannot be known without a figure : sometimes it shows plenitude of blood ; especially if the veins be high, if gravel or red sand appear at the bottom it shows the Stone in the reins, kidneys, or bladder. If the urine be of a light sandy colour, and somewhat thick, it shows great cold taken, and oft times it turns to an ague, and the urine be flinty and somewhat thick, it threatens worms in young people, and consumptions in elder ; but if the urine be green or black coloured it usually shows death to ensue, also if the urine be of a sad brown colour it threatens death, I question not but that Authors have largely and learnedly written hereupon, to whom I shall [refer myself ; for] I do seldom trust, or rely upon my judgment herein, neither do I administer any Physick thereby for the Astrological, Sympathetical and antipathetical way of administering Physick cannot be done without a Figure, for the strength and weakness of the Planets afflicting and afflicted must first be discovered ; those who are well versed in the Art of *Astrology* need no urine, for I myself oft times, when the urine has been brought in a stone bottle have described what kind of urine it was, and how coloured by my figure, more especially in acute griefs, when the time of decumbiture or first falling ill have been known.

Concerning the casting forth of Devils out of such, who are possessed, with the true way and manner how to do it according to the Author's experience and performance thereof, with some observations, whereby to know whether they are possessed or no.

THe occasion which first moved me to undertake the casting forth of Devils was as follows. One Goodman *Alexander* a Turner by trade, living at *Basing-Stoke* in the County of *Southampton* had a Daughter, who was not only perplexed with very strong fits, which usually took her every day near the same hour, every fit lasting above twelve hours, being very terrible to behold, during which time with many shrieks and cries, and through extreme torment she was brought so low, both in body and Spirit, that she could not move or wag any part of her body or limbs from the middle downward ; her Father told me he had spent much money upon several Doctors and others but they could do her no good, whereupon hearing by some, what great cures I had done, he came and told the what her condition was, as I have in part related, desiring me to undertake the cure. I desired to know at what hour and time her fits usually began, which he told me, according to which time I erected a Scheme, and according to the Rules of *Astrology* in this book else where expressed, I found she was either bewitched or possessed : Her Father was very earnest with me to undertake the cure, and I could not blame him, she having been in this condition, above twelve months ; and besides he made his bargain so, that if I did nor effect the cure, I was to lose all my pains and charges upon which, agreement being made ; the Maid was brought to my house, whereupon observing and taking notice of her kind of fits, and having made same trial upon her by way of questions, and her answers, for she could not say, or once name God, Jesus Christ, or Deliver us from Evil, or the like but that immediately she would be tormented, falling into strange fits : whereupon I told her Father, that she was possessed by the Devil, and that it would be impossible to cure her, except the Devil were first cast forth ; I also advised him to get one godly Minister or other to try what he could do by his means, and devotion ; whereupon, and not before he told me that he had done that already : For the Minister of the Parish, whose name was Mr. *Webb* one reputed to be very honest, godly and Learned man did undertake to do it : and came to his house two several times to that purpose, but could not prevail ; not withstanding he spent about three hours time in trial thereof at his first coming ; yet he was forced to desist : but withal, told her father, that at the next coming he would be better prepared, and accordingly he did come the second time, but could not prevail then neither, during all the time that he was in action about this business the Maid was extremely tormented, it being as before near three hours before he ended, who then said to her Father, *Lord have mercy upon me I cannot do it, wherefore I advise you to look out farther, peradventure you may meet with one or other who may have strength of faith, and a gift to do it, and likewise to cure her distemper.* I confess, when I heard by her Father, what the Minister had done, I began to be somewhat daunted, but when I considered that it would much reflect upon my reputation to send the Maid home again uncured ; and further considering, that by Prayers, and strength of Faith it might be done ; more especially, where it pleased God to give any one that gift, which gift is obtained by Prayer, and strength of Faith : I also further considered, that both before and since Christ's time Devils were cast forth out of such who were possessed, as appears by the answer of our Saviour Jesus Christ to the Jews, who taxed him, saying, *He casts forth Devils through Beelzebub the Prince of Devils.* If I say our Saviour cast forth Devils through *Beelzebub, by whom did your Fathers cast them forth* : by which words it appears that the *Jews* had done it before Christ's time : And further tells them, *That a Kingdom divided cannot stand &c.* Considering these reasons aforesaid, according to the method hereafter expressed I undertook and through God's blessing perform this great work, to whom be ascribed all honour, Power, and Glory, with Thanksgiving, for ever more, *Amen.* Before I proceed to set forth the way and manner, how I did through God's blessing perform this great work, I conceive it will be necessary to say somewhat concerning the trial of the Patient, whereby to know, whether they are possessed or no, which is as follows, If they can without stop or starting say the Lords Prayer : also pronounce God, Jesus, Christ and likewise say, I defy the Devil and all his works, and other such like Godly expressions : then 'tis probable they are not at that time possessed : and then you must try them again at another time : for as we find in Scripture, them are some which are possessed at certain times, and at other times the Devil leaves them. But as concerning this Maid in question, the Devil did never forsake her, from the time he first entered into her. Also some are possessed with Devils which speak within them at certain times, as instance, this Maid was : others are possessed with dumb Spirits which will not speak, nor yet many times suffer the Patient to speak, nor yet to pray, or pronounce God, Jesus Christ, the holy Trinity, or any other such like expressions, for fear of being tormented with fits. I have cast forth of both kinds, out of such who were possessed, as shall be shown in order I shall first begin with this Maid in question, whose fits began about nine o'clock at night, and lasted until eight o'clock the next morning; during which time she was most sadly afflicted, making many kinds of noises, as sometimes crying, screeching, howling, also sometimes using strange actions and gestures of her body, as twisting, and twining herself about, sometimes crawling about the room with many other strange passages. Now from eight o'clock in the morning until noon, she would resolve all questions whatsoever, and give true answers to them as have many times been proved, more especially, if propounded by her Mother, for she did not desire to talk with any other body except by accident ; during this four hours they usually put many questions to her, as sometimes asking, what became of any one that was dead, whether they went to Hell or to Heaven, and she would instantly resolve them ; and so far as they could guess she answered truly ; for those who had been evil livers she would tell all their faults and misdemeanors, and how they lived, and died, and what disease, and where they were buried likewise : such who were godly persons she would say they went to heaven and point upwards, although they were such whom she never saw or knew. Also she would tell the names

Casting out a devil

of any one's Father, or Grandfather, (although they were strangers) and where they lived and died, and of what disease. She would likewise during the time aforesaid resolve any question of theft, whereof they had many trials, I shall instance one example, upon a market day, one chanced to lose a sack of Corn out of the Market : The man having pitched his sack down in the Market, and went away to set up his horse, but before he returned, his sack of Corn was stolen, and nobody could tell what became of it : at length understanding that this Maid could tell anything that had happened for any time past, he went to the said Goodman *Alexander* the Father of this Maid, desiring him to use the means that so his Daughter might discover what became of his Corn, whereupon, the Mother of this Maid desired her to tell this man, who had his Corn, and what became of it, and where it was at that instant : This Maid said, that one, calling him by his name, had the Corn, and had set it under his stairs ; the man that stole it, was a Porter that used to carry burdens in the Market, more especially Corn, when it was bought or sold. The man who lost the Corn went presently to the place aforesaid, where he had his Corn accordingly. I could instance many more such passages, but I suppose this one is enough for satisfaction herein. Now as concerning the way and method by me used, in casting forth of both kinds of Devils, or evil Spirits before mentioned ; I shall relate as follows, (there are three principal causes or things considerable in casting forth of Devils, *viz.* Prayer, Faith, and the special gift of God thereupon, for except that you find that your Faith is strong, it's in vain to undertake this business :) First, you must heartily pray that God would be pleased to give you this great gift, and to strengthen your Faith, and to enable you to perform this great work : this was the substantial matter of my Prayer, as for matter of form I had none ; the room being made in readiness so close as I could, I made a fume of three substantial matters, or things which were Solary, which number three I conceived to be a most choice select number for many persons, and is attributed to the *Sun*, its the number of the blessed Trinity, it's also the number of time, *viz.* past, present and to come ; also I considered, that the three wise men brought gifts to Christ, *viz.* Gold, Frankincense, and Myrrh, which gifts are all of a Solary quality and virtue, and are under the dominion of the *Sun*, whereupon I made choice of the two latter, *viz.* Frankincense and Myrrh, but instead of Gold I took Rosemary with these I made the fume, which I continued until the work was ended : I also oft times gave the Maid of the distilled waters of Marigolds, Rosemary and Angelica, or such like Solary plants, being all three under the dominion of the *Sun*, and gathered at the right planetary hours, when I first began, I laid my hand upon the Patient, but finding that she together with the Devil began to strive and so to get from me, she being marvellous strong, yet I held fast, and desired her Father (who was by me all the while I was about it) to help me, which he did, but for the most part I held her myself having gotten her at the best advantage I could : I often prayed and repeated these words following, *viz.* by this high and mighty Power and Name *Tetragrammaton* and in the name of the blessed Trinity, Father, Son, and holy Ghost, I charge, and command the Devil and unclean spirit to come forth of this Maid, and to depart from her in peace, and not to molest or trouble her any more ; after this, when I saw that the unclean Spirit would not come forth, I said three several times, *In the name of Jesus of Nazareth I charge thee to come forth*, yet not withstanding, (as yet) the Devil would not come forth : the truth is, I find that all Devils or evil Spirits, when once they are gotten into the possession of any one will be very unwilling to come forth of their habitation ; more especially, when they have been long settled in the body : I often gave the Patient of the distilled waters before mentioned, and then prayed again as at the first ; I also repeated those words before mentioned oftentimes, resolving not to give over until the Devil was enforced to leave her, and during the space of above two hours I continued sometimes in Prayer, and between whiles repeating the words over before rehearsed ; at length the Devil came forth but invisible, with a great cry and hideous noise raising a sudden gust of wind, and so vanished, doing no harm either to her Father (who was present all the while) nor yet to myself, or any part of the house : her Father seemed to be very fearful, and sat trembling, (and truly I do not much blame him for I believe he was never present at any such business before) but I cheered him up so well as I could, biding him fear nothing, and willed him to trust in God not doubting : the truth is, when I saw him so fearful I willed him to depart, telling him, that except he found that his Faith was strong, and he thoroughly resolved to endure the danger, cries, noise, and trouble of it, he might unhappily interrupt me when I was most busy ; for he knew by what the Minister had done before, that we should have some struggling : but his answer was, that what ever came of it he was resolved to live and die with his Child, rather than fail ; whereupon I went on with the work, but before I had half done my task, he hearing and seeing how grievously his Daughter was tormented, his Spirits and Faith began to fail him, desiring me by all means to desist, and give over ; but I being very earnest with him, and telling him of his breach of promise, and using some arguments to him, and telling him that except he would either sit still and not any more interrupt me, or otherwise depart the room, I would not meddle any further in the Cure, whereupon he resolved to endure it, and promised me once more that he would be silent until I had finished, which accordingly he did perform ; immediately after the Devil left her the Maid began to speak, and the fits never troubled her any more ; and within a few weeks after, with Diet-drinks, baths and ointments, this Maid was perfectly recovered both of her health, and limbs ;

notwithstanding, for a year past, she could not move from the middle downwards, her limbs being useless, and of no strength, except during the time of her fits, and then sometimes she would be very strong, and at othertimes seemingly dead, foaming at the mouth, sometimes she would shriek, cry, and groan, sometimes crawl about the room, as in part I have before related : I shall relate one passage more which happened constantly in the time of her fits, there was always brought to her three pins and but one at a time, at the receipt thereof she seemed to rejoice and smile, saying, *ah* and then presently she would put the pin into her mouth, which when her Father and Mother perceived, they would instantly get it from her, fearing she would choke herself with it ; sometimes they were much troubled to get it from her, for she would be very unwilling to part with it ; they showed me a box near full of them for she had three brought her every night during twelve months ; and that night when I cast the Devil forth of her she had two brought her in my presence but no more ever afterwards ; also 'twas observable, that during the time that I was employed about this business, there was seen by my people and servants three Women to walk about the house, and more especially, near the Window where I was employed, which women her Father did judge were three suspected witches, who had spoken some words, and were afterwards prosecuted by the Maid's Father, one of them died, as I was informed at the Prison in *Winchester*, and what became of the other two I know not, for I never enquired more after them.

I shall now proceed to set forth the way and manner how I cast forth a dumb Spirit out of one who was possessed, as follows.

THat which confirmed me and others of this Maid now in question, of her being possessed of a Dumb Spirit, was in regard that she could not say or once name God, Jesus Christ, nor yet endure to pray, or suffer any one else either to pray, or repeat any Sacred words or expressions, but that immediately she was tormented, and sometimes would fall down dead : This Spirit would not answer to any question as the other speaking Devil did, not yet suffer the Maid : in her fits she was always dumb and silent, her fits usually began about five o'clock in the morning, and lasted four hours, during which time she would not utter one word, but would sometimes leap about with her arms and legs like a Frog, sometimes she would play cop-head, over and over ; sometimes with all the might she had, she would knock her head against the Bed-post or Wall, which was nearest. Also being in a Chamber she would strive to get to the stairs that so she might throw herself down. Now the way which I used to cast forth this dumb Spirit, was as follows, In the first place the room being made so close as I could with convenience, I made a fume of such solary ingredients as is before expressed ; which fume I continued all the time I was in this action : the time which I took to cast forth this dumb Spirit, or Devil, was between the hours of nine and twelve o'clock upon the Sabbath day : the prayers which I used, was according to what I have already related in casting forth the speaking Spirit ; and likewise I oft repeated the same ways as aforesaid. But this dumb Spirit would not come forth until the third Sabbath day : Notwithstanding, I was near three hours every time in action, & during all the time I was employed in this business, she would be much afflicted ; upon the third Sabbath day between the hours aforesaid, this dumb Spirit came forth in a kind of vomit, no shape or form of any thing appearing, after which, by diet drink and ointment made of Planetary herbs, antipathetical to the afflicting Planet, she was soon recovered and never had any more fits after the third Sabbath day before mentioned. *Note*, That dumb Spirits are far more difficult to be cast forth than those which speak : and that was the only reason why I took the benefit of those hours upon each Sabbath day, it being the usual hours of Prayer in all Churches, and Congregations.

I know there are some foolish people, who being ignorant of the Scripture, that do, and will judge unrighteously concerning this great work, unless they are convinced, and truly I need not use any other arguments than what we find written by the holy Evangelists and Apostles, as first, the answer of our Blessed Saviour to the *Jews*, as is before mentioned. Secondly, we find that our Saviour gave that special gift to his Apostles and Disciples ; and without question to all other believing Christians, who may through strength of Faith do it ; as appears in *Mark* Chap. 16 *ver*. 17. And when the Apostles told our Saviour *that they did forbid some who undertook to do it*, our Saviour said, *forbid them not, &c.* But to such who presume to do it who wanted Faith and did not Believe : nay, although they used the very words of the Apostles, yet the Devil would not obey, nor yet be commanded forth by them : as you may find in the 19 *Chap*. of the *Acts* of the Apostles, there you shall find, that one *Sceva*, a *Jew* had seven Sons who were exorcists, or Conjurers, these following *Paul* and the Apostles, and hearing the words which they used, assayed to do the like, presuming to cast forth a Devil out of one who was possessed, saying, *I adjure you by Jesus, whom Paul Preached to come forth*, but the evil Spirit answered and said, *Jesus I know, and Paul I know, but who are ye* ? *And the man in whom the evil Spirit was, fell upon them, beat them and tore all the clothes from their backs*, and without question put them into a great fright, for we find, that they all seven ran out of the house wounded, and naked, and, glad (I warrant you) that they escaped so, this act of theirs was noised abroad, and also known throughout all the City of *Ephesus*, and fear fell on them all, insomuch, that I believe never any *Jew* dared attempt any such thing afterwards to this day ; for St. *Mark* says plainly, *These Signs shall only follow those that believe in Christ Jesus* : in his name shall they cast out Devils ; wherefore, to those, who believe not in Christ Jesus, it plainly appears they shall not do it. And whosoever does, or shall undertake this business, his faith and belief must be strong without doubting, otherwise he may fail in the performance, for although some ceremonies may be used herein as I have before related, yet without God's special blessing upon the words, ways, and means used, together with strength of Faith, believing, no man can prevail herein, as plainly appears by those seven Exorcists, or Conjurers aforesaid.

Concerning all kinds of Agues, and quotidian Infirmities, the Astrological way of Cure.

THere are three kinds of Agues, *viz. Quotidian, Tertian*, and *Quartan* ; of all which kinds I have Cured many : And to my knowledge and best remembrance I never failed where I have undertaken, I once cured a Woman who had a *Tertian* Ague nine years, being brought so low therewith, that she was not able to go without help ; she had without question as she told me, taken many things for it, but without success. I find there are many recipes by Authors set forth in Print, but I could never find any certainty in them : I dare say, there are so many ways invented for the curing of Agues, as there are people sick of them : there can be no certainty in curing any of these kinds of Agues, or daily fits, or griefs, except it be done by the Rules of *Astrology*, for many reasons, for some are afflicted under the Planet *Saturn* and then their fits will be most of cold : others are afflicted under *Mars*, and then their fits will be most of heat : and some are afflicted under both Planets, *viz.* *Saturn*, and *Mars*, and then their fits will be never equal both in cold and heat. *Secondly*, sometimes the afflicting Planets are weak in the Heavens, and sometimes strong, which must be considered in the cure. *Thirdly*, the Age and Complexion of the Patient must be taken Notice of. *Lastly*, you must by a Figure discover whether any *Witchcraft* or *Sorcery* has been wrought upon the Patient, or from what natural cause the sickness began. I shall now briefly discover the reason of each kind of Ague, or *Quotidian* Infirmity, and then set forth the way of cure as follows, I shall begin with the *Quotidian* Ague, which usually assaults the Patient daily, near one and the same hour, at which time as also in *Tertians* and *Quartans* the sick usually is troubled with wind and cold watery phlegmatic matter settled at the stomach, which at the first beginning of the fits causes a shivering, after which follows a feverish burning hot fit ; and I find, that not only the *Quotidian* Ague, but also there are many other infirmities, as Apoplexies, Convulsions, Palpitations, Risings in the Throat and Stoppings at the Breast and Stomach and some kinds of Evils which daily begin to afflict the Patient near the same hour : Now upon observation upon all these kinds of daily Agues or Infirmities before mentioned I constantly find, that the Sign Ascending, at or near the beginning of each fit, together with its Lords exactly personates the sick, and without doubt was their proper Ascendant at their Birth, by virtue of which Ascendant, together with the sixth and twelfth houses, and their Lords afflicted, I always discovered the grief, with its cause and termination : the truth is, except a Figure be set for either the time of Decumbiture, or first fit, or some other strong fit, there can be no true discovery made from what cause it began, and if the true cause be not known, there can be no certainty in cure ; for although the *Moon* in acute and the *Sun* in Chronic sicknesses by the Planets afflicting, generally discovers each distemper with its cause, yet in these particular infirmities as Quotidian griefs before mentioned, I find by experience, that the fits have constantly kept their course, and have been very strong when neither *Sun* or *Moon* have been afflicted, wherefore it appears, that the sign or Constellation under which the Patient was born (which Sign we usually call the Ascendant) wholly reflects upon the Patient both at the beginning and duration of their daily fits aforesaid ; and truly I find even as in *Quotidian Agues*, and other infirmities aforesaid, so likewise in Evils ; The Ascendant usually personates the sick, more especially when the fits are usually near one hour, or at the time when the Patient undergoes any strong pain or torment more than other ; for such is the subtlety of the Devil, that he knowing each body's Ascendant, can thereby the better instruct the *Witch* how to frame the Image, that so it may thereby work the stronger upon the Patient when the Sign ascends, and by that means the *Witch* may by the rules of *Astrology* be the more easily discovered, and oft-times are thereby detected, for its well known to many, that in a Philosophical way when a Talisman is framed for the destruction of vermin, as instance, the *Scorpions*, the way to make it is when the Sign *Scorpio* Ascends, &c.

Concerning the Tertian Ague.

THe *Tertian* Ague usually keeps one hour, as the *Quotidian* Ague does, only there is one day's respite between, now I find, that in *Tertian*, and *Quartan* Agues the *Moon* is much to be regarded, for, from the time of the first fit, which may probably be called the time of decumbiture, the place of the *Moon* in the *Zodiac* must be observed, and so by account according to the Critical Figure of sixteen equal parts (what the Critical Figure is, and how framed, I have shown more at large elsewhere) each fit answers to the Intercedental, Judicial, and Critical days and times, and so the second fit makes the Intercidental time ; the third fit the Judicial time, the fourth, the second Intercidental time, the fifth the Crisis, and so you may go round the *Zodiac* : after which the grief is Chronic, and may unhappily continue a long time, if not cured. *Note,* that notwithstanding by account, according to the Critical figure, of its equal parts there is but 21 *deg.* 30 min. allotted for two days motion of the *Moon,* whereas usually she moves 24 *deg.* at the least ; yet if we consider the beginning, and duration of each Ague fit, and likewise what Degrees are allotted to the Orbs or Influence of the *Moon* ; it will sufficiently satisfy those Degrees in question. Now as in the *Quotidian* Ague so in this, If you fear Sorcery or Witchcraft, and make doubt of the true cause of the Ague, a figure set for the time of the first, or any other fit, more especially when its very strong will be needful, which to do I have shown elsewhere.

Concerning the Quartan Ague.

THe *Quartan* Ague usually gives two days respite between every fit and as in the *Tertian* Ague so in this, the *Moon* has a special Influence upon both, all Ague fits comes sometimes sooner, and sometimes later, according as the *Moon* is swift or slow in Motion more especially, when evilly aspected of the infortunes. The Degrees of the *Moon's* Motion which by account are numbered between each *Quartan* Ague fit are 45 *deg.* making a *Semi-quartile* aspect to the place she was in at the decumbiture, or first fit ; and so the second fit may be called the Judicial time. The third fit the Crisis or Mortal time consisting of 90 *deg*. making a square Aspect to the place she was in at the decumbiture aforesaid ; in *Quartan* Agues the Critical figure is divided but into eight parts; the Intercidental time being left out as useless, in regard the fits are at such known distance from each other ; It seems *Hypocrites* and *Galen* never used any other division in their times : But since we find by experience, that at the Intercidental time many have departed, as I have shown elsewhere, especially in perperacute griefs. All *Quartan* Agues are under the Dominion of *Saturn*, and usually, if the *Moon* be evilly aspected of him, at the time of any *Quartan* Ague fit, then it will be more violent and strong ; although these *Quartan* Agues are usually of long continuance, yet they are seldom mortal ; the reason is (I judge) because there is usually two days respite between every fit, whereby nature has time to rally up its forces against the encounter. What I have written concerning Agues and *Quotidian* infirmities is from my own daily Practice and Experience, for I never met with any Author either in Print or by Manuscript which showed the reasons of each kind of Ague, nor yet any certain way of cure : I shall in the next place set forth the certain way of Cure, as follows.

The way to Cure each kind of Ague according to the Rules of Astrology : *there being no certainty in any other way, as I have oftentimes experienced.*

IN the first place (according to the Rules in this book elsewhere expressed) you must erect a Scheme either for the time of the first fit if that may be had, or for any other strong fit ; you must be careful so to vary the Ascendant, that it, together with its Lord may exactly personate the sick, for if you take a wrong ascendant which you may easily do for many reasons, as first the difference in Clocks, secondly, the swiftness or slowness of the *Moon's* motion, thirdly some men and women being strong hearted will not yield to lie down in bed so soon as others who are more weak and faint hearted, *&c.* wherefore if you fail in the Ascendant no true judgment can be given, except in ordinary, natural, acute, and chronicle griefs, or where there is no suspicion of Sorcery or Witchcraft, for then judgment may be given by the *Sun* or *Moon* afflicted, as is shown elsewhere : when your Scheme is Erected, and the Figure Radical as aforesaid, you must take notice, whether the Lord of the Ascendant, or first house be in the twelfth house or whether the Lord of the twelfth be in the Ascendant, or whether one Planet be Lord of the Ascendant, and twelfth, and an infortune, or if the Lord of the twelfth afflict the Lord of the Ascendant, or whether the Lord of the twelfth afflict the *Moon*, in acute griefs which are under a month's standing, or the *Sun* in Chronic griefs, then you may conclude that the *Quotidian* fits of any kind and likewise the *Tertian* and *Quartan* fits of any Ague are more than natural ; and that either Fascination, Witchcraft, or Sorcery, have been wrought upon the Patient ; such is the subtlety of these wretches, that many times they are not mistrusted much more discovered, except by the Rules of *Astrology*, described as I have shown elsewhere, and who more bold and forward to visit and frequent Neighbours, and ofttimes are employed both for Nurses, and tenders upon those whom they have bewitched and yet not mistrusted, and were there no ways to afflict them, there could be no cure wrought upon such whom they daily visit or are employed as tenders upon : For by their wretched ways, they would soon infect them again : *Example*, Once a Friend and Neighbour of mine, after she was delivered of her Child fell into strange fits, whereupon, some thought she had taken great cold, others thought, some one thing and some another, at length her fits grew so strong, and the Woman so weak, that her Husband thought at every fit she would have departed, whereupon, he was advised to come to me ; but to prevent his coming, the Tender or Nurse being a lusty young Hussy would needs persuade him to send her with the Water, which he did, at her first coming she seemed to be very merry and jocund always laughing, I asked her why she was so merry, considering her Dame was so bad, she told me for no harm, I believe she thought to have fooled me, as she had done others (but she was greatly mistaken) for having viewed the Urine, I demanded of her to tell me whether she had any fits, and when her first fit began, which she readily told me, not thinking that I could thereby discover her Villainy ; I quickly found by the Figure, that Sorcery or Witchcraft had been wrought upon the sick, and by a Female body, much resembling her person ; for either the Lord of the twelfth house, more especially of that is the afflicting Planet or the Sign where the *Sun* is, usually personates the Witch ; whereupon I told her that I could send no answer by her, in regard, I must first speak with her Master ; at which answer she seemed some what daunted, but replied, she would speedily send him, and so went away, but when she came home, she clean contrary to my message told him, that she had order to gather herbs and make his Wife Diet-drink, and none but she must give her any thing to help her ; whereupon, the man marvelling much at this message came to me on purpose to know the truth, why none but she must be trusted and brought his Wife's Brother with him whereupon I told him, what I found by the Figure, his brother presently replied, that to his knowledge, both her Mother and Grandmother were both suspected for Witches, and one of them died in *Reading Goal*, being Committed by the Justice with intent to bring her to Trial : having made this discovery upon her, I advised him speedily to put her away, and to take another Nurse or Tender who was of better repute, which he did ; after which, by such ways and means as were agreeable to her distemper, according as I have declared at large elsewhere, she was soon recovered. I shall now proceed to set forth the *Astrological* way of Cure, for there is no certainty in any other way (notwithstanding, sometimes the Patient is cured by other means, as I shall declare in the sequel) more especially when the original of the fits, either of Agues, or other *Quotidian* infirmities before mentioned, be from Sorcery, or Witchcraft, for then in the first place, you must by the rules beforegoing endeavor to afflict the Witch, otherwise she will continually renew the grief so fast as you cure, more especially where the Witch is not suspected. *Secondly*, you must be careful that such herbs which are used for the Cure, be gathered at the right Planetary hours, with the numbers of herbs according as they are attributed to each Planet : what herbs are to be used herein, together with the time of gathering, administering, and the numbers of herbs are set down elsewhere. The true way of curing all kinds of Agues, and other Quotidian fits must be by antipathy, not omitting as in these, so in all other Cures, to take a select number of herbs to fortify the heart and vital Spirits. There are four things considerable to be done in curing all kinds of Agues, besides the afflicting of the Witch, in case of Sorcery, or Witchcraft, *First*, Diet-drink ; *Secondly*, Cataplasms laid to the hand wrists. *Thirdly*, a vomit, to be given at the coming of the fit : *Fourthly*, to let blood if the Ague has been of long continuance. *Fifthly*, to cause the Patient to wear one or more Solary Plants : The way which I always used, is as follows, having by the Figure found under what Planet the Patient is most afflicted, as instance *Mars* then take herbs under *Venus* ; if under *Saturn*, then take herbs under *Jupiter* ; if both *Saturn* and *Mars* afflict, as sometimes 'twill fall out, then let your herbs be under *Jupiter* and *Venus* ; but if *Saturn* and *Mars* be strong in the Heavens, and more strong than the fortunes *Jupiter* and *Venus*, then their own herbs will do it ; always provided, that one of the smallest numbers of herbs under one or both the fortunes, together with herbs of

The Astrological way to cure Ague   177

the *Sun* be used together with the rest ; but if the infortunes be weak, then the smallest number attributed to them, and the greater number of the fortunes together with a select number of herbs under the *Sun* will do it, for the Diet-drink you may together with the herbs, aforesaid, add Raisins, Currants, Liquorice, Aniseed, Sweet fennel-seed, or Coriander seed, to make the Diet-drink nutritive, as also more pleasant and good to expel wind : the Diet-drink is made by way of decoction and given to the Patient three times a day *viz*. morning, afternoon, and night : I have cured many only by Diet-drink and herbs, suitable as aforesaid, laid to the hand-wrists, made up by way of Cataplasm : The herbs which you lay to the hand-wrists must be shred very small and pounded in a Mortar with Raisins and white Salt, you may add a little *Venus*-Turpentine to make it hold together, you must use the quantity of two walnuts, it must be laid on hot and bound fast to the hand-wrist: if the Patient does not mend after one or two fits trial, then you must give the Patient a vomit, just when the fit begins as follows : Take one dram of *Stibium* more or less according to the strength and age of the Patient, beat it into a very fine powder with a Pestle and Mortar, then warm a quarter of a pint of white wine and put the powder into it, keep this in a glass twenty four hours and shake it often, and when the Ague is ready to come put forth the wine into so much new milk, but leave the dregs behind and give it the Patient blood warm and let them take posset drink after every vomit, if the Patient does not amend after one or two fits trial, then you must let the patient blood, for after the Patient has been afflicted above a Month 'twill get into the blood also, if need require you must give the Patient another vomit, more especially, If the Ague have been of long continuance, and I have sometimes been enforced to let blood more than once ; you must still give them diet-drink until they are well ; If you heed well what I have written you need not doubt of curing all kind of Agues, although of long continuance, as also from what cause soever it had its beginning. By the Rules aforesaid I cured a Woman who had a *Tertian* Ague nine years, as aforesaid.

Another way whereby to Cure all kinds of Agues Astrologically ; together with other infirmities which are in the Blood or Vital Spirits, as I have oftentimes proved, is as follows.

WHen you let the Patient blood, take a small thimble full of Sympathetical powder, and the like quantity of the powders of such herbs which are suitable to the cure, as aforesaid, mix them well together and put a small quantity of the blood into this powder, and be careful that it take no cold, for both the powder and blood must be put together warm, and let the Patient wear it next their skin, you must be careful that the herbs used, be gathered at the right Planetary hours according to their numbers as formerly mentioned, by this way, I have cured both Agues and other infirmities.

There it yet another way whereby to cure Agues.

THis way is performed only by a certain writing which the Patient wears. Now whether there were any such words passed between our Saviour and the *Jews* as the writing mentioned who can tell, for without question there were many memorable actions, things, and words, said, and done by our blessed Saviour which are not recorded in holy writ, and we find words in Scripture, tending to that purpose : The words are as follows.

When Jesus went up to the Cross to be Crucified the Jews asked him, saying, art thou afraid, or hast thou the Ague ? Jesus answered and said, I am not afraid, neither have I the Ague. All those which bear the Name of Jesus about them shall not be afraid, nor yet have the Ague, *Amen, sweet Jesus, Amen, sweet Jehovah, Amen.*

I have known many who have been cured of the Ague by this writing only worn about them ; and I had the receipt from one whose Daughter was cured thereby, who had the Ague upon her two years.

Concerning several kinds of madness, with the true, Astrological *way of Cure, as follows.*

I shall not enter upon any large discourse hereof nor yet take notice of Authors, who without question have written Learnedly hereupon. My intent being only to write what I find by my own daily Practice and experience herein : according to which I find, that there are several causes of madness, and several kinds of madness I mean in relation to their actions and behaviour, whilst they are in this condition : First, concerning the Cause, for except it be known, it's impossible, except by accident to work a cure, which for to find, you must erect a Figure, either for the time of the first fit, or any other more than ordinary strong fit, and to be sure, so to vary your ascendant, that it together with its Lord may exactly personate the sick, and then by the Rules of Art, examine whether the grief be Natural or otherwise, from Witchcraft or Sorcery : if Natural, then from what original cause, as whether from love, loss of honour, friends, estate, or any other, more than ordinary vexation, and such like ; for then the distemper will be wholly in the Animal and vital spirits, for we may be assured, that whatsoever the external or internal senses do comprehend, which proceed from the brain : the Vital spirits which proceeds from the heart do immediately put into action be it mirth or sorrow : in curing these kinds of madness, you must heed the Complexion and Temper of the Patient ; for as in Drunkenness, so in Madness, you will assuredly discover their Elemental, Qualities, and Natural Conditions : If Choler abounds, then they will be violent in their Actions and very apt to quarrel. If they are by nature Sanguine, then they will be inclined to mirth, as singing, dancing, and the like. And such who are by nature Melancholy, and Mad, usually are given to sadness, sighing and much silence, seldom pleased. And those who are by nature Phlegmatic mad, are usually sluggish and idle, not caring to do any thing, except forced thereto, and much given to sleep, they will lie in bed two or three days together, if not disturbed. The way to cure all these kinds of distempers before mentioned must be by decoctions, made of such herbs under such Planets which are antipathetical to each several Complexion before mentioned ; not omitting ointments to the heart and brain, and fumes to the head, if the brain be moist and suffumigation if dry. If the Patient has been long distempered, then 'twill get into the blood, and then 'twill be convenient sometimes to let them blood ; and then if you take a small quantity of the Sympathetical powder and mix it with so much Powder of the herbs proportionate for the Cure, it will mightily help forward the cure : you must order it and wear it as directed in the curing of Agues. There are several other kinds and causes of madness as follows, sometimes height of blood will ascend up to the head and so disturb their brain, which will cause madness, the curing whereof is by oft letting blood, and diet drink made suitable by Antipathy to their Complexion, as aforesaid ; for if we should apply herbs which are by nature hot, although good in general for the brain, to a Choleric mad body, it will rather increase, then mitigate their fury, but in all cures you must ever remember to fortify the heart and vital Spirits: the Sympathetical powder in this

Madeness by reason of bound in the body   181

kind of madness, mixed and ordered as aforesaid, is most proper; the truth is, this kind of madness is easily cured by any drug-Doctor, for their general way is to cure by bloodletting, and purgation, which kind of Physick is proper for this distemper. There is another kind of madness which comes by being costive & bound in body of which I have cured many, and I always found by the Figure, that the chief significators of the distemper were in earthy signs : for the time being, these who are taken in this condition will be as mad, as any according to their natural Complexion, be it Choler, Sanguine, Melancholy, or Phlegmatic ; at the first they will be ill only in head and stomach, but after some time it will make them light headed, and forgetful ; and by reason of that great stop in Nature's Course ; it will more and more cause inordinate Vapours to ascend up to the head and brain, and at length bring madness, insomuch, that they are not able to discover their own condition nor yet their friends ; I have known some who have died in this condition, before their grief was perfectly known, or at least, were so far gone that Doctors could not help them. I had once a Maid (who was a Farmer's Daughter, living in the Parish of *Goring* in the County of *Oxon*) brought tied and bound fast in a Cast with Cords, who was only mad by reason of this condition, her Friends not knowing what she ailed, some thought it might be through Love, others thought she was either bewitched or possessed ; some thought one thing, and some another : the truth is, she looked very ghastly and wild but being by nature of a Sanguine Complexion, she would whoop, holler, sing, and dance day and night if she might be suffered : having by a Figure discovered the cause of her distemper, I bargained with her Father what to have for the cure, I quickly with suppository and glister brought her to stool, and within three days she grew sensible and quiet, and in a week was perfectly recovered. I have known sometimes that an afright has caused madness ; in this condition applications must be chiefly to the brain, not omitting Diet drink, made suitable by antipathy to their Complexion : I have known some Females who have been mad only by the stop of their monthly Course ; the cure is by herbs proper to help such infirmities, as you shall find in this book. I have known some women, who have fell mad after they have been delivered of their Child ; occasioned sometime from great cold taken, or disorderly diet and sometime by Witchcraft (as I have already declared, occasioned by the Tender, or Nurse ;) for their bodies being open and weak, any infirmities may the easier be wrought upon them by such wretches, and yet the cause undiscovered and the Patient many times dies.

The worst kind of madness that I know is occasioned from Sorcery or Witchcraft ; and I believe there are multitudes of this kind in *Bedlam*, and elsewhere, that lie many years in this condition ; for except the Witch's power be taken off and stayed, it's in vain to administer Physick ; more especially, where the Witch sometimes may have admittance to come to the Patient : others may perhaps be possessed, and then the Devil must be cast forth ; for (as I have said already,) except the true cause of each kinds of madness be discovered, it's impossible to cure without a Miracle, except by accident ; now to cure this kind of madness which comes from Witchcraft : In the first place, you must by the Rules of Art, endeavour to afflict the Witch, and then by herbs antipathetical to the afflicting Planet and complexion of the Patient you must make Diet-drinks, Ointments, and Glisters, not omitting some ingredients suitable, as Figs, Raisins; Currants, Liquorice, Aniseeds, or any other seeds good to expel wind, *&c.* & sometimes when the body is bound, which most mad people are very subject to ; you must make choice of such herbs amongst your Numbers which are Purging and loosening. *Note* that I always found in my Practice, that the afflicting Planet and Complexion of the Patient were usually one, as instance, Choleric people are commonly afflicted of *Mars*, and Melancholy under *Saturn*; for such is the subtlety of the Devil, and the Witches, that they strike most upon that humour whereto they find the nature of men and Women most prone, and apt to receive impression.

If these Rules which I have inserted, be well observed and followed, there is no one mad body whatsoever, but may (through Gods blessing) be recovered : to my knowledge I have not failed these many years where I have undertaken ; not withstanding, some whom I have cured have been mad many years : but I must needs say, the longer they are mad before a right means is used, the more difficult the cure is and somewhat the more time it will require to perfect their cure : For according to that saying in Philosophy, *Custom produces a second Nature*, &c.

FINIS.

To all such who are Students, and well-wishers to this most excellent Science of Astrology,

I Presume, that no sooner are these following Books come forth, but some will be ready to say, What needs this Treatise, since we have so many books of this nature extant, written both so Learned and Copious even in our own Language that one would think, nothing more could be written of this Subject? but yet we know, that in all Arts and Sciences whatsoever, no man can so curiously and exactly write of any matter or thing, of what Nature soever, but that something might be added thereunto ; and were it but only a confirmation of what has been written formerly by other Authors, yet it's but reasonable, that such persons who have been Practitioners and Students in this Art, should likewise have liberty to write their Knowledge and Experience herein : And although in general we keep close to one entire Method and Rule, as in our Introduction appears, compared with others, even as with young Scholars, so in this Science, there must be beginning or entrance at the first, after which, each industrious Student and Practitioner may increase in knowledge, and so make further progress and discoveries herein ; and having attained thereunto some perfection, may do well to communicate their knowledge to others, that so this Art may continually be enlarged : we find that in all Ages this Art has increased, by means of those Worthies who have been Students and Practitioners therein, whose Books are extant of this nature : I confess, in some material matters and circumstances I differ from many Authors, yet I keep close to the Principles of Art, giving sufficient reasons for what I write ; those that read my Books, being compared with other Authors may follow that way and method (which by trial) manifests itself to be most effectual : I do not intend by this my writing, in the least, to disparage other worthy Authors, but do highly praise and extol those excellent Works written by our Learned and Ingenious Country-men, who have taken much pains in Demonstrating the Art ; only as I have already said, where there is a Continuance of Practice each ingenious person may without doubt add something to the increase of knowledge ; and I question not, but that each Practitioner and young Student will gain somewhat by my Labours herein. And as for such who are well learned in this Art, although my writing may not add much to their knowledge herein, yet in point of wisdom and love to the Art and Artist I presume they will take what I have written in good part, and pass by my failings (if any) with silence : But as to the envious, they shall not much trouble me, considering their persons will be sufficiently rewarded, as being to themselves most destructive. But to such who are loving and true lovers of the Art, I wish a blessing upon their Studies and that they may increase in knowledge, *Vale.*

Appendices
(added by the Editor of the 2010 edition)

List of herbs

This list of herbs was derived from the catalog of cures, pgs. 83–109, and was used to check spelling and consistency. I include it here in the hopes readers may find it of use. – Editor

A: adders-tongue, adonis flower, agrimony, alcanet, alehoof, alder tree, Alexander, allheal, almonds, aloe, amber, amphier, anemony, anet*, angelica, aniseed, apples, apricot, archangel, archangel blossoms, aromatical reed*, arrach, arrowhead, arsmart, arsmart root and seed, artichokes, asarabacca, ash, ash-tree, ash-tree bark, ashen-keys, asparagus, asparagus roots, asphodel, avens, avemony*

B: balm, balm-apple, balsam, barberries, barley, barley flower or meal, barrenwort, basil, bayberries, bayes (bay leaves), bay tree, bean, bear's breech, bears ears, bear's-foot, beech, beech-tree, beets, bellflower, betony, bezar-tree*, bilberries, bindweed, birch-tree, birds-eye, bird's-foot, birthwort, bishop's weed, bistort, bitter-sweet, black-alder, black alder tree, black-cherries, black hellebore, blackthorn leaves, blites*, bloodwort, bluebottle, blue pimpernel, borage, borage-blossoms, box, boxthorn, brambles, brooklime, broom, broom-blossoms, broom-buds, broom-rape, bryony, bugle, bugloss, bulleys, burdock, burdock-root, burgundy pitch, burnet, butcher's-broom, butterburr, butterwort

C: cabbage, calamint, calendine, caltrop, camels-hay, cammock, camomile, camphire, campion, capers, caraway, caraway-seed, carduus, carnations, catmint, cattail, cedar, celandine, centaury, century, charlock, cherry-tree gum, chervil, chestnuts, chickweed, cicely, cinnamon, cinquefoil, cinquefoil-roots, clary, cleaver, clivers, cloudberries, clove-gillyflowers, clowns-all heal, cockle, cockshead, coffee, colewort, coltsfoot, columbine, comfrey, comfrey roots, coriander, coriander-seed, costmary, couch-grass, cow-parsnip, cowslips, juice of crabs, crabtree, cranesbill, cresses, crosswort, crowfoot, cuckoo flower, cuckoopint, cucumbers, cudweed, cullians*, cumin, currants

D: daffodil, daisy, damask-roses, dandelion, danewort, darnel, dates, dry dates, hot dry dates, devil's-bit, dill, dittany, dittany of Crete, dock, dock bastard*, dodder, dodder of thyme, dog's-mercury, dragons blood, dropwort, ducks-meat, dwarf-elder, dyer's-weed

E: eglantine, *Egyptian*-thorn, elder, elder-buds, elder-flowers, elecampane, elmpeel, elm-tree bark and leaves, endive, eryngo, eye-bright

F: fennel, fennel-root, fennel-seed, sweet-fennel-seed, fenugreek, fern, feverfew, figs, fig-tree, figwort, filberts, filipendula the roots, flax, flaxweed, fleawort, flower-de-luce roots, flower-wort, fluellin, foxgloves, foxstones*, frankincense, herb-frankincense, fraxinus, friar's-cowl, fumitory, furzbush-flowers

G: galingale, galls, gall of an ox, garden-tansy, garlic, germander, gillyflowers, ginger, glasswort, goat's-beard, goldenrod, gooseberries, gourds, goutwort, grapes, grasie*, gromwell, ground-ivy, ground-pine, groundsel, guaicum

H: hacraper*, hart's tongue, hartwort, hawkweed, haws, hazelnuts, hazel-tree, heart's-ease, heartwort, heath, hedge-mustard, hellebore, hemlock, hemp, hemp-seed, henbane, herb mercury, herb-terrible*, herb true-love, herb twopence, hog's-fennel, holly, holly-berries, honeysuckles, honeywort, hops, horehound, horsemint, horseradish, horsetail, horse-tongue, houndstongue, houseleek, hyssop

I: inner yellow bark of black elder, ironwort, ivy, ivy-berries

J: Jack by the hedge, jessamine, Jesuit's bark, Jews ears, Jews-thorn, juniper

K: kidneywort, knapweed, knotgrass

L: lady's bedstraw, lady's mantle, lady's thistle, larkspur, laserwort, laurel, lavender, leeks, lentils, lesser centaury, lettuce, lilly, limes, liquorice, liverwort, loosestrife, lovage, lungwort, lupine

M: mace, madder, maidenhair, mallows, mandrake, marigolds, marjoram, marshmallows, masterwort, mastic-tree, maudline*, meadowsweet, medlars, medlar-stones, melilot, melilot flower, melons, mezereon, milkwort, millet, mints, mirabilan, mistletoe, moonwort, moss, mother of thyme, motherwort, mouse-ear, mugwort, mulberries, mullein, mustard, myrobalans, myrtle

N: nep, nettle, nightshade, nutmeg

O: oak, inner bark of oak, oats, oil of green wheat, oil of

trotters, oil of wheat, oil-pulse, olives, olive-tree, one blade, onions, oranges, orpine, Osmund-royal, water-Osmund, ox-eye, oxlips

P: parsley, parsnip, peach, peach flowers, peach leaves, peach-tree, pearmain, pear tree, pellitory, pellitory of the wall, pennyroyal, peony, pepper, periwinkle, pilewort, pimpernel, pine, pippin, pitch, plantain, ploughman's-spikenard, pockweed, polypody, polypody of the oak, pondweed, poppy, potatoes, powder of steel, primrose, privet, prunes, hot prunes, hot stewed prunes, purple wort, purslane

Q: quick-grass, quinces

R: radish, ragwort, red archangel, red-beans, red beet-root, red corral, red-nettles, red pebble-stone, red poppy, red-roses, red wild campions, rhubarb, ribwort, rice, rind of oak, rocket, *rosa solis*, roses, rosemary, rosemary flowers, rose-wood, rue, rupturewort, rye

S: saffron, sage, Saint *James*-wort, Saint *John's* wort, Saint *Katharine's* flower*, Saint *Peter's* wort, samphire, sanicle, sandalwood, satirion, savin, savory, saxifrage, scabious, sciatica-cresses*, scorpion-grass, scurvy-grass, sea-dogs grass, sea green, sea-holly, self-heal, sene, sengreen, sensitive herbs*, services, sheep's dung, shepherd's-needle, shepherds-purse, skirrets, sloes, smallage, snails, snakeweed, sneezewort, soapwort, sorrel, sour apples, southernwood, sowbread, sowthistle, spearmint, sperage, spikenard, spignel, spinach, spinage, spleen-tree, spleenwort, spurge, staggerwort, starwort, stitchwort, stinking arrach, stinking gladdon, stinking gladwin, storax, strawberries, succory, summer savory, sundew, swallow-wort, sweet-apples, sweet basil, sweet marjoram, sweet-maudlin, sycamore

List of herbs

T: tamarind, tamarisk, tamarisk tree, tamarisk-wood, tansy, tarragon, thorow-wax, throatwort, thyme, toadstools, tobacco, toothwort, tormentil, trefoil, turbith, turnip, young turnip-leaves, turpentine, twayblade

V: valerian, vervain, vetch, vine, vine-leaves, vinegar, violets, violet-flowers, leaves, and footstalks, violet roots, vipers, viper's grass, viper-wine, virgins-bower

W: wake-robin, wall, wall-gillyflowers, walnut, watercresses, water-fern, water-germander, wayfaring-tree, wheat, wheat-meal, white-beets, white-lilly root, white poplar, white poppy, white roses, white-wine, red-wine, whortleberries, wild carrots, wild citrus, wild-tansy, winter-cresses*, winter-gillyflowers*, winter savory, woad, wolf's-bane, wood-betony, woodbine, woodruff, wormseed, wormwood, wound-tree

Y: yarrow, yew

Z: zedoary

The pre-Copernican World

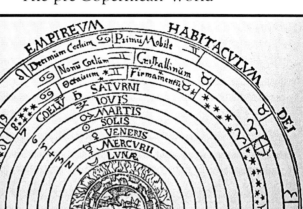

Around the outside, the words, *Coelum Empireum Habitacuium Dei et Omnium Electroum*: Heaven, the Supreme Abode of God and the Elect (i.e., Angels).

Inside the circle, ten concentric heavens. The outermost, the 10th heaven (*Decimum Coelum*), is the Primum Mobile, or First Cause, aka rapt motion. We know this as the Earth's daily rotation on its own axis. Inside it are the 9th (*Coelum Crystallinum*: Sphere of Crystal), the 8th (*Octavium Firmamentum*: Sphere of the Starry Sky), and then the spheres (in order) of Saturn, Jupiter, Mars, Sun, Venus, Mercury and the Moon. At the very center, the *Sublunary World*, i.e., the Earth.

Use pages 194-195 in conjunction with the text on lost items, strays and fugitives (pgs. 153-159), with reference to planetary positions in the spheres (higher and lower), and rulerships, terms and faces. — *Editor*

A Table of the Essential Dignities of the Planets according to Ptolemy

Azimene Degrees

Aries: none
Taurus: 6, 7, 8, 9, 10
Gemini: none
Cancer: 9, 10, 11, 12, 13, 14, 15
Leo: 18, 27, 28
Virgo: none

Libra: none
Scorpio: 19, 28
Sagittarius: 1, 7, 8, 18, 19
Capricorn: 26, 27, 28, 29
Aquarius: 18, 19
Pisces: none

Temperament

Extracted from
Astrological Practice of Physick
by Nicholas Culpeper

    Infallible signs to discern of what Complexion any person is whatsoever.

Signs of Cholerick men

    The cholerick man for the most part is little, and short of stature ; which happens (as I suppose) either by reason of the fewness of vapours and fumes engendered ; or else, because that the radical moisture whereby the virtue nutritive and vegetable is sustained, is by the operation of strong heat and drynesse drawn to the centre, and there partly consumed ; as fire (of whose nature is choler) attracts moisture to itself, and dries it up, so that the superficial and extreme parts stretch not in length, neither wax big, or fat, because of defection of natural moisture, (as in aged persons in whom radical moisture is decayed) grows no more : and his skin is rough and hot to touch, & his body very hairy, their colour is between yellow and red, with a certain glittering like fire ; such persons soon have beards, and the colour of their hair is red, or auburn. As touching their conditions, they are naturally quick-witted, bold, unshamefaced, furious, hasty, quarrelsome, ireful, fraudulent, stout, arrogant, courageous, graceless, cruel, crafty, and inconstant ; light in moving, jesters, mockers, watchful, and flatterers, &c. their eyes little and hollow. Also the virtue of concoction in them is very strong, insomuch that he may digest more then he has appetite for ; his pulse is swift and strong, his urine yellow, and thin in substance ; as touching their digestion, they are often costive, they dream of fire, fighting, and anger, of lightning, and dreadful apparitions of the air, by the means of hot and dry fumes and vapours ascending from the stomach into the head, which trouble the brain and virtue imaginative.

Signs of Cholerick Melancholy man.

Cholerick melancholy men, are higher of stature than cholerick, because violent heat in them is more remiss and slack, whereby fumes are the more engendered, and radical moisture the less wasted ; yet they are little and lean of body, because of drynesse, with skin rough and hard, meanly hairy, and temperate in feeling ; their colour is palish, drawing towards a brimstone colour, for in it is seen a little skew of yellowishness ; they have not beards so soon as cholerick men, and the colour of their hair is reddish, or light auburn. And touching the conditions, or natural inclination of such persons, they are not altogether so pregnant witted, bold, furious, quarrelsome, fraudulent, prodigal, stout, and courageous as cholerick men ; neither so graceless, inconstant, flattering, swift, and scornful as they ; yet they are suspicious, fretful, nigerdish, and more solitary, studious, and curious than cholerick and retain their anger longer. The virtue of digestion in such persons is meetly strong, and their pulse lesser and slower then in cholerick persons ; their Urine is yellow and thin, and they dream of falling from high places, of robberies, murders, harms proceeding of fire, fighting, anger and much like.

Signs of a Melancholy Cholerick man.

Melancholy Cholerick men are tall of stature, by reason that natural heat is feeble, and thereby many fumes are engendered, but they are little and slender of body, because of dryness, therefore their skin is rough and hard, and cold to touch : they have but very little hair on their bodies, and are long without beards, by means of cold which stops the Pores, and suffers not the matter whereof hair is engendered to come forth : much superfluity in the nose ; their colour is pale, shadowed with a little negritude, or darkness. And concerning their conditions, they are gentle, given to sobriety, solitary, studious, doubtful, avaricious, shamefaced, timorous, stubborn, fretful, pensive, constant, and true in action, with a deep surmise, and slow wit, with obliviousness ; their hair is brown and thin, their digestion feeble, and less than their appetite, the pulse little and slack, their urine subcitrine and thin ; and they dream of falling from high places, fearful dreams, and sundry varieties.

Signs of Melancholy men.

Melancholy men are mean of stature, and seldom very tall ; for excess cold binds the substance, and suffers it not to stretch in length ; and although melancholy be dry in temperature, yet they are little, and slender of body, the occasion (I imagine) of excess cold, by means whereof much superfluity is engendered, which somewhat alays the dryness, for melancholic men are full of Flegm, and rumatique matter. Their colour is duskish, and swarthish pale, their skin is rough and cold to touch ; they have very little or no hair on their bodies, and are long without beards, yea, sometimes beardless ; the colour of their hair is duskish ; as touching their conditions, they are naturally covetous, self-lovers, fearful without cause ; pusillanimous, solitary, careful, lumpish, seldom merry or laughing, stout, stubborn, ambitious, envious, fretful, obstinate in opinions, of a deep cogitation, mistrustful, suspicious, vexed with dolours of the mind, and dreadful imaginations (as though they were infested with evil spirits) and are very spiteful, curious, squeamish, and yet slovens, high-minded, and very majestic in behaviour, and retain their anger long ; the virtue of concoction in them is very feeble ; yet they have very good appetite to their meat. Their Urine is palish and mean in substance, and they dream of fearful things, terrible visions, and darkness.

Signs of Melancholic Sanguine man.

Melancholic sanguine men are higher of stature then melancholic ; for in them natural heat is temperate ; wherefore fumes and radical moisture are meanly engendered, whereby they are meanly big ; fleshier, and firm of body ; their colour is after a darkish red, their skin neither hard nor rough, but temperate in heat and softness, and not very hairy ; they have beards about 21 years of age ; and touching their conditions, they are more liberal, bolder, merrier, less stubborn, and not so pusillanous, solitary, and pensive, as melancholic persons, nor so vexed with dreadful imaginations as they are : also they are gentle, sober, patient, trusty, merciful, and affable ; and to conclude, for as much as this complexion is temperate in quality, so likewise it is boon in conditions ; for virtue is a mean between two extremes. Their urine is of light saffron colour, and mean in substance ; their pulses are temperate in motion ; they have pleasant dreams, and many times respondent to truth ; and their digestion is meanly strong.

Signs of a Sanguine Melancholic man.

Sanguine Melancholic men are mean of stature, with bodies well compact with reins and arteries ; fleshy, but not fat ; they have skin meetly smooth, and hot in feeling, and are somewhat hairy, and, soon have beards ; the colour of their hair is dark auburn, their cheeks red, shadowed with gluteal colour.

Their conditions are much like to a sanguine man's, but they are not altogether so liberal, merry, and bold, for they have as it were a spice of the inclination of melancholy persons. Their pulses are great and full, urine yellow and mean in substance, with dreaming of deep pits, wells, and such like ; their digestion is indifferent.

Signs of a Sanguine man.

 Sanguine men are of a mean form, their bodies well composed, with larger limbs, and fleshier, but not fat ; with great veins and arteries, smooth skins, hot and moist to touch, the body hairy, and soon bearded ; their colour is white, intermixed with redness in the cheeks ; their hair for the most part is brown. And touching their conditions, they are merry, liberal, bountiful, courteous, bold enough, merciful, trusty, faithful, and of good behaviour ; a little thing will cause him to weep, and when that is done, no further grief sticks to their hearts ; which is contrary to melancholy men, for they cannot weep, although it be in a matter that concerns them near, but yet their cogitation thereof is imprinted in their hearts. The sanguine man has good appetite, and quick digestion ; his urine is yellow and thick, his pulse great and full, and dreams of red things, and pleasant conceits.

Signs of a Sanguine Phlegmatic man.

 Sanguine phlegmatic men are higher of stature then Sanguine, because more superfluities are engendered in their bodies, and are of substance much like to Sanguine ; their hair is flaxen, or light auburn, their colour is like red, but not intermixed as Sanguine are ; as touching their conditions, they are less liberal, sadder, and not so bold as Sanguine and not so hairy ; their urine is subcitrine, and mean in substance, their pulses moderate, with good appetite, and digestion indifferent ; they dream of flying in the air, and falling down from some mountain, or high place into water, or such like.

Signs of a Phlegmatic Sanguine man.

Phlegmatic Sanguine men are mean of stature, and somewhat gross of body, with a smooth and soft skin, and cold in touching ; their bodies are hairy, and long without beards ; their hair is light yellow, or flaxen, plain and smooth ; their colour is neither white nor red, but mean between both ; of conditions, neither very merry, nor much sad ; not liberal, or covetous ; not much bold, not very fearful, &c. The virtue of digestion in them is somewhat slack, and lesser then their appetite, their pulses are low and little, with dreaming of sundry fables.

Signs of a Phlegmatic man

Phlegmatic men are shorter of stature, for although much vapours and superfluity is engendered in their bodies, yet by means of coldness the substance is bound and stayed from stretching in length ; nevertheless moisture deals itself in breadth, and makes them gross and fat. Their veins and arteries are small, their bodies without hair ; they have little beards, and their hair is flaxen ; their colour whitish, with smooth skin, and cold to touch ; As concerning their conditions, they are very dull, heavy, slothful, sleepy, cowardly, fearful, covetous, self-lovers, slow of motion, shamefaced, and sober. In them the virtue of digestion and appetite is feeble, (through defect of natural heat) their pulses are little and slow, and their urine pale and thick ; with dreaming of water, &c.

Signs of a Phlegmatic Cholerick man.

Phlegmatic cholerick men are tall of stature, and not so big and fat as phlegmatic, and are more hairy, and sooner have beards ; their hair is light auburn, in which some show of yellow, and are temperate in feeling ; And touching their conditions, they are nimbler, bolder, and kinder than phlegmatic, and are not so drowsy, and sluggish as they are, but merrier, and quicker witted ; Their face for the most part is full of freckles, and their colour white, shadowed with yellowishness : their appetite and digestion is indifferent ; their pulses are moderate and full, their urine subcitrine and mean in substance, dreaming of swimming water, or snow or rain.

Signs of a Cholerick phlegmatic man.

Cholerick phlegmatic men are mean of stature, firm, and strong of body, and neither fat nor lean, with great legs, and their skin hairy, and moderate in feeling, their hair is yellowish, and their colour the same ; their conditions are not much different from cholerick men, but they are not altogether so furious and bold as they, neither so prodigal, and guileful ; for flegm does somewhat allay the heat of choler ; their digestion is perfect, their pulse swift, and their urine like Saffron and thin, with dreaming of battles, strife, lightning, and hot water.

Glossary

A. Intensity and frequency of disease

Intensity:

The shorter the disease, the more intense. A plague-type disease typically ran its course in two days or less, usually resulting in death.

Ruled by the Moon:

Acute: Diseases lasting from a week, up to a lunar month. From the square / first crisis, up to the fourth.

Peracute: Diseases lasting three to four days, or 45° (semi-square) of the Moon's travel, or up to the first Judicial Time.

Perperacute: Diseases lasting less than two days, or 22° 30' (semi-semi-square) of the Moon's travel, up to the first Intercidental Time.

Ruled by the Sun:

Chronic: Diseases / infirmities which have lasted more than a month.

Frequency: (See also pages 216-8.)

Quotitian Agues produce daily fits or seizures.

Tertian Agues produce fits every other day. They respond to Intercidental, Judicial and Critical times.

Quartan Agues produce fits every fourth day. They respond to Judicial and Critical times. Commonly believed to be malaria.

B. Individual terms, glossed

This was assembled from several sources and includes terms which Blagrave did not use in his text, but which are contemporary to him. I believe these definitions to be correct, but there are differences of opinion, and modern authorities are sometimes mistaken. This list also includes terms which I was unable to define, try though I did. — *Editor.*

Agrippa, Cornelius — German magician, occultist, theologian, astrologer, and alchemist. Born September 14, 1486, died February 18, 1535.

Agues — Malaria. A condition with alternating periods of chills, fever and sweating. *See page 203, and pages 215-6.*

Anareta — Killing planet.

Apoplexy — A rupturing of a blood vessel. The most common are cerebral hemorrhage (stroke) and pulmonary.

Apostem — Abscess.

Azimene degrees — See the list on page 195.

Bedlam — Blagrave used its proper name, Bethlem. The Bethlem Royal Hospital of London, since 1347 famous as a mental institution.

Berm — Possibly a kind of sugar, or a yeast.

Bites of mad dogs — Rabies.

Black bile — Symptoms are depression, hypochondria, melancholy, etc.

Black jaundies — Said by some to be hepatitis, but Cornell specifically states dark brown or greenish-black skin discoloration.

Blood corrupted — Cornell gives synonyms as, impure, foul, heavy, coarse, stagnant, poisoned, toxic, filled with waste materials, etc. He says it is primarily a Jupiter affliction.

Blood distempered — Similar to corrupted, above.

Blood putrefied — Presumably an intense form of corrupted blood. There is no reason to think Blagrave is referring to scabs.

Bloody flux — Dysentery, e.g., a disease in which the flux or discharge from the bowels is mixed with blood.

Bole armeniac — An astringent clay-like earth formerly from Armenia.

Bound in body — Constipated.

Bubo — An inflamed, tender swelling of a lymph node, especially in the armpit or groin. The bubonic plague was a severe form.

Burgundy pitch — Spruce resin.

Calenture — A fever caused by exposure to great heat, possibly sunstroke. Affected sailors sometimes imagined the sea to be a green field, and to throw themselves into it.

Cataplasm — A poultice, or a medical dressing consisting of a soft heated mass of meal or clay that is spread on a cloth and applied to the skin to treat inflamed areas or improve circulation etc.

Carbuncle — An acute inflammatory nodule of the skin caused by bacterial invasion to the hair follicles or sebaceous gland ducts. A boil that has more than one focus of infection.

Cardiac passion — Heart attack. Cornell says palpitations and spasms.

Catarrh — A head cold, or, in general, inflammation of the mucous membranes, including those of the eyes, with discharge. This can have a daily cycle.

Celandine water — According to Culpeper, water prepared from the common or greater celandine, also known as swallowwort. Also known as salandine water.

Chin cough — Whooping cough.

Choler, Choleric — One of the four humors of ancient and medieval physiology, thought to cause anger and bad temper when present in excess. Associated with yellow bile, summer, fire and gall bladder.

Climacterial Periods — Every seventh year in a nativity (some say every seventh and ninth), from the Moon, as by transit, the Moon squares her position every seven days, which means that by secondary progression, she squares herself every seven years. When evil directions coincide, the result is said to be potentially fatal, especially in the later Climacterial periods. (*Adapted from de Vore*.)

Cliches/clinches of the arms — The inside of the elbow.

Collick/Colic — Acute abdominal pain, especially in infants.

Combust, combustion — Blagrave judges this to be when a planet is within 7°30' of the Sun.

Concupiscence — Lust.

Concoction — A sauce of various ingredients.

***Consideratis, considerandi**s* — With the necessary considerations.

Consumption — Tuberculosis, phtisic, any wasting disease, not limited to the lungs.

Convulsions — Uncontrollable spasms.

Coral tree — Any of various mostly deciduous trees or shrubs of the genus Erythrina in the pea family, native to and widely cultivated in warm regions, having trifoliolate leaves, showy red or orange flowers, and pods containing often brightly colored seeds.

Cordial — Serving to invigorate; stimulating.

Costive — Constipation.

Critical day or time — In a decumbiture chart, when the Moon has travelled 90°, which it does in about a week, from the position it held at the time of the decumbiture. By extension, 180°, 270° and 360°. *See also* Intercidental, *and*, Judicial.

Crudity — Raw foods.

Dead Palsie — General paralysis, perhaps as a result of stroke.

Decoction — An herbal preparation made by first mashing, and then boiling.

Decumbiture — A chart drawn for the time the patient takes to his bed. In modern terms, when the ambulance comes.

Deflux — A downward flow of humors or fluid matter, as from the nose in catarrh.

Degrees first, second, third, fourth — Levels of intensity. In terms of disease, a "first degree" illness would be mild. A fourth degree illness would be fatal. This classification, which was common in Blagrave's day, is still used for burn wounds.

Directions, from page 157 — London is traditionally ruled by Gemini, Oxford by Capricorn, Reading by Virgo, and Scotland by Cancer. Taken from medieval lists of rulerships of cities and countries. There are horary directional techniques that can be used for other locations.

Distemper — To upset the balance of the humors, generally referring to most any ailment.

Dropsical humor — A general swelling, from fluids.

Dropsy — Edema, or swelling, especially in the lower legs.

Ebullition — A sudden, violent outbreak.

Eversion — Turned outward, turned inside out. Eversion of the ventricle refers to the ventricle in the larnyx.

Exulceration — An ulcer, or sore.

Falling evil — Epilepsy.

Fancy — Faculty of forming mental images.

Fascination — In witchcraft, a form of induced hypnosis.

Fistula — An ulcer opening on to the skin. When arising from injuries suffered during childbirth, can result in uncontrolled discharge of urine or feces. Women with such injuries were typically spurned.

Flank — The side of a person or an animal between the last rib and the hip.

Flux — Diarrhoea or mucous discharge, intensifying towards sunset.

Formentation — Hot, wet compress or bandage.

Fraxinus — Of the ash tree.

French or Spanish Pox — Syphilis. One notes with wry amusement how this disease always bears the name of some other country.

Frenzies — A state of violent mental agitation or wild

excitement, temporary madness or delirium.
Frowardness — Stubbornness.
Fume — To treat with fumes, smoke, or vapors.
Fundament — Buttocks or anus.
Galen — A Greek doctor who lived from 131-c.200 AD. Holden says his astrological writings are "apocryphal", which might have been a surprise to Blagrave.
Gall — Bile.
Gargareon — Also known as Uvula. The spongy mass that hangs down at the back of the throat.
Glister — All references say, "glitter", which is clearly not correct.
Gout — A disturbance of uric-acid metabolism occurring chiefly in males, characterized by painful inflammation of the joints, especially of the feet and hands, and arthritic attacks resulting from elevated levels of uric acid in the blood and the deposition of urate crystals around the joints. The condition can become chronic and result in deformity.
Great heat (in the back) — Kidney infections.
Greensickness — A form of anemia common in young women, accompanied by menstrual disturbances and a greenish skin color. Also known as Chlorosis.
Grief — To Blagrave, any physical hurt or harm, any disease.
Grissels — Cartilage.
Guiacum — A shrub or tree native to the Caribbean.
Haly — Haly Abenragel (d. after 1037), court astrologer to the Tunisian Prince al-Mu'izz ibn Badis. Best known for his comprehensive book on astrology, *The Outstanding Book on the Judgments of the Stars*.
Hams — The buttocks.
Haunch — The hip, buttock, and upper thigh in humans and animals.
Heart strings — Angina pectoris, or the tendons or nerves formerly believed to brace the heart.
Hectic — A fever that fluctuates during the day.

Hemorrhoids — Veins liable to discharge blood. Piles refer specifically to veins in the anus.
Huckle-bone — The hip bone.
Humor — One of the four basic fluids in the body. They are: Black bile, yellow bile, blood and flegm.
Hylegical places, five — 1st, 11th, 10th, 9th and 7th houses.
Hypochrondiac melanchololy — Extreme depression.
Hypocrites — Alternative spelling of Hippocrates.
Iliac-passion — Jane Ridder Patrick describes this as "a disease characterized by severe gripping pain, constipation, vomiting of faecal matter and spasm of the abdominal muscles." The iliac region are the flanks.
Implead — Legal: To bring action against.
Imposthume — An abscess.
Inappetency — Lack of desire.
Incurvating — Crooked, not straight.
Ingurgitation — Gulping.
Intension — Stress.
Itch, the — Scabies.
Intercidental time — In a decumbiture chart, when the Moon has travelled 22°30', which it does in about 42 hours, from the position it held at the time of the decumbiture. By extension, any 22°30' of travel that is not otherwise defined as a Judicial or Critical time. *See also* Critical, *and*, Judicial.
Judicial time — In a decumbiture chart, when the Moon has travelled 45°, which it does in about three and a half days, from the position it held at the time of the decumbiture. By extension, 135° and 315°. *See also* Critical, *and*, Intercidental.
King's evil — Scrofula, tuberculosis of the lymph glands; so called from a notion which prevailed, from the reign of Edward the Confessor to that of Queen Anne, that it could be cured by the royal touch.
Lambative — A lincture, a medicine taken by licking with the

tongue.

Lask — Diarrhea or flux.

Left ear phrenzies —

Limbeck still — Limbeck refers to alembic, which is a still.

Lohoch — See Lambative.

London Dispensary — The Encyclopaedia Britannica says the London Dispensary was founded in 1696, which is clearly wrong, as Blagrave was using it 30 years before.

Lord of the day — The Sun rules Sunday, the Moon rules Monday, Mars rules Tuesday, Mercury rules Wednesday, Jupiter rules Thursday, Venus rules Friday, Saturn rules Saturday.

Lord of the hour — The planet ruling the hour of the day. See Planetary hours.

Lues Veneria — Syphilis.

Malapert — Arrogant.

Matrix — The uterus.

Mediety — Half.

Melancholic — One of the four humours, cold and dry. Associated with black bile, autumn, earth and spleen.

Melancholly blood — Cornell says the Moon afflicted in Virgo, by the Moon itself.

Membranes — Of the brain.

Miseraicks — The veins of the mesentery, or peritoneum, the membranes that hold the small intestine in place.

Mother fit — A choking sensation said to be caused by the womb's rising.

Moveable signs — Cardinal signs: Aries, Cancer, Libra, Capricorn.

Mutatis, mutandis — With the necessary changes.

Neatsfoot oil — Extracted from the shin bones and feet of cattle.

Necromancy — Communicating with the dead in order to predict the future, a form of magic.

Noli me tangere — Touch me not: A name formerly applied to several varieties of ulcerous cutaneous diseases, but now only to Lupus exedens, an ulcerative condition of the nose.

Palsy — Uncontrollable trembling, paralysis, weakness.

Paps — The breasts.

Paroxysm — A violent, excruciating seizure of pain.

Partile aspect — Any aspect which is less than one degree from exact. See Platic.

Peccant — Morbid.

Pellicle — A thin skin or film.

Peregrine — Said of a planet which has no dignities in the degree and sign in which it is located. See the table on page 195.

Pestilence — A serious, widespread, but not especially contagious affliction.

Phlebotomy — Opening a vein, bloodletting.

Phlegmatic — One of the four humours, cold and moist. Associated with phlegm, winter, water, brains/lungs. Having or suggesting a calm, sluggish temperament; unemotional.

Phrenetic — Wildly excited or active; frantic; frenzied. (Variation of frenetic.)

Phthisis — Any illness of the lungs or throat, such as asthma, cough, or, in extreme cases, tuberculosis.

Physic — A purge.

Pipes — Bronchial tubes.

Pipkin — A small earthenware pot.

Pippin — A crisp tart apple having usually yellow or greenish-yellow skin strongly flushed with red.

Pissing disease — Diabetes.

Planetary hours — Planetary, or astrological, hours are one-twelfth of the time from sunrise to sunset, and one-twelfth of the time from sunset to sunrise. They are never of sixty minutes duration except at the equinoxes, and so must be calculated for one's precise latitude and longitude (see Editor's Preface). The first hour of the day starts at sunrise and is ruled by the planet which rules the day itself. For example, the first hour of Sunday is ruled by the Sun. The rulers of the following hours are in this order: Venus, Mercury, Moon, Saturn, Jupiter, Mars, and then, repeating, the Sun, &c. If this is followed, it will be seen that the first hour of Monday is ruled by the Moon, which rules the day.

Plaster — A medical dressing, bandage.

Platic aspect — Any aspect which is not exact to the degree, or which is outside the normal orbs allowed. See Partile.

Pleurisy — Inflammation of the membrane that covers the lungs and lines the chest cavity. It is sometimes accompanied by pain and coughing.

Polypus — A polyp, or small tumor, usually in the nose, throat, ear, or rectum.

Posset — A hot drink made from milk curdled with ale, wine, or other liquor, often with sugar, spices, and herbs.

Praecordiacs — Vessels of the heart.

Priapism — Prolonged or painful erection of penis or clitoris.

Privy Parts — External sex organs.

Probatum est — It has been proved.

Ptisick — Tuberculosis.

Pulvis sanctus — A ready-made powder, the name probably covers a number of different recipies. One was to combine one pound each of aloes, senna, ginger, and cream of tartar.

Purgation — Purging the body by the use of a cathartic to stimulate evacuation of the bowels.

Purples — Poor circulation in the extremities.

Pushes — Eczema, pustules.

Quartan — *See page 203, and pages 216-8*

Quinces — Hard yellowish fruit with sharp flavour.

Quinzies — Tonsillitis.

Quoad capax — According to capacity.

Quotitian — *See page 203, and pages 216-8*

Red Choller — An itchy, burning skin disease.

Reds — Menstrual flow.

Reins — The kidneys.
Repletion — A state of excessive fullness. Gluttony.
Rheum — Mucous discharge from membranes of nose, throat or mouth.
Rickets — A softening of the bones in children, due to a lack of vitamin D, or lack of calcium.
Ridgebone — Backbone.
Risings in the throat — Nausea.
Roman vitriol — Copper sulfate.
Running of the reins — Gonorrhea.
St. Anthony's Fire — Either erysipelas, an acute skin infection, or ergotism, from eating grain infected with ergot fungus.
Sal gem — Sal ammoniac.
Sallet oil — Either sweet oil, or goose or duck liquor (rendered goose or duck fat).
Salt flegm — Cornell refers to salt rheum, which he says is chronic eczema.
Sanguine — One of the four humours, warm and moist. Associated with blood, spring, air, liver. Confidant, enthusiastic.
Scab, the — Scurvy.
Sciatica — Pain along the sciatic nerve usually caused by a herniated disk of the lumbar region of the spine and radiating to the buttocks and to the back of the thigh.
Science — Art, skill, or expertness, from the application of laws and principles.
Scirrhus tumour — One that is hardened.
Scurf — Scaly or shredded dry skin, such as dandruff.
Secundine — Part of the afterbirth.
Sedge — Grasslike and rushlike herbs found in marshes.
Seed — Semen.
Semi-quaratile — 45°.
Semi-semi quartile — Half of half of a square: 22°30'.
Shingles — Herpes zoster.
Sic in aliis — And so in other cases.

Siccity — Dryness.
Soil — As in, "where soil is laid": manure.
Spettle — Spittle
Spirit of wine — Another name for brandy.
Squinzies — Diptheria, as opposed to tonsillitis/quinzies.
Stibium — Antimony.
Strangury — Slow, painful urination.
Sublated — Literally, to negate or deny. In relation to pulse, weak or none?
Suffumigation — Fumes, mist or strong odors delivered by means of evaporation, as by means of alcohol.
Surfeit — Overindulgence leading to nausea.
Swoon — Faint, black out.
Swounding fits — Possibly delirium.
Sympathy — A relation between parts by which a condition in one induces an effect in the other.
Terrene — Of the earth.
Tertian — *See page 203, and pages* 216-8
Tetters — Herpes, ringworm or eczema.
Throat-almonds — Adenoids.
Throat kernals — Tonsoliths, from chronic cryptic tonsils.
Tragacanth, gum — Made from goat's thorn, or locoweed.
Trotter — The feet of goats, pigs, lambs, or any cattle.
Turning of the ventricle — The ventricle in the larnyx, the laryngeal sinus.
Tympanic — Referring to the eardrum.
Uvula — Also known as Gargareon. The spongy mass that hangs down at the back of the throat.
Venery — Indulgence in or pursuit of sexual activity.
Ventricle — Not chamber of the heart, but rather part of the larnyx. *See* Turning of the ventricle.
Venus turpentine — Probably Venice turpentine, which is made from the larch tree.
Verjuice — The juice of unripened grapes.

Via combusta — The "burning way". 15 Libra to 15 Scorpio. Immanuel Velikovsky had an interesting theory as to the origin of the term.
Virtue — Strength.
Water-gruel — A thin, watery soup.
Wen — A large cyst, often seen on the neck.
Whelk — An inflamed swelling, such as a pimple or pustule.
Whites — Vaginal discharges.
Wind cholic — Gastric distress, flatulence.
Windiness in the veins — Cornell says a Gemini disease.
Yellow jaundies — Jaundice.

I found the following on-line as I was about to send the book to the printer. It is too good to ignore. It is from Smith's Family Physician, by William Henry Smith, and was published by John Lovell in 1873. — *Editor's note.*

Ague, Intermittent Fever

When the cold fit comes on every twenty-four hours, it is called a Quotidian; when there is a space of forty-eight hours between the attacks, it is called a Tertian; and when it appears on the first and fourth days, it is called a Quartan. That under the tertian type is most apt to prevail in the spring, and is the most common form of the disease. The quartan is the most obstinate and dangerous, being chiefly prevalent in autumn and winter. The quotidian is more likely than the others to assume the continued type.

The tertian Ague generally makes its attacks in the forenoon, the quartan in the afternoon, and the quotidian in the morning. The quartan, which has the longest intervals between the fits, has the longest and most violent cold stage, but, upon the whole, the shortest paroxysm. The hot fit of the tertian is comparatively the longest. The quotidian, with the shortest interval, has at the same time the longest paroxysm.

An Ague fit is composed of three distinct stages: the cold, the hot, and the sweating stage.

A person who it on the brink of a paroxysm of Ague, experiences a sensation of debility and distress about the region of the stomach; he becomes weak, languid, listless, and unequal to bodily or mental exertion. He begins to sigh, to yawn, and stretch himself; and soon he feels chilly, particularly in the back, along the course of the spine; he grows pale, his features shrink, and his skin gets dry and rough. Soon the slight sensation of cold, first felt creeping along the back, becomes more decided and more general: the patient feels very cold, and he acts and looks just as a man does who is exposed to intense cold, and subdued by it; he trembles and shivers all over; his teeth chatter, sometimes so violently that such as were loose have been shaken out; his knees knock together; his hair bristles slightly, from the constricted state of the skin of the scalp; his cheeks, lips, ears and nails turn blue; rings which before fitted closely to his fingers become loose; his breathing is quick and anxious; his pulse frequent some-

Extract from Smith's Family Physician, 1873   **217**

times, but feeble; and he complains of pains in his head, back, and loins; all the secretions are usually diminished; he may make water often, though generally he voids but little, and it is pale and watery; his bowels are confined, and his tongue is dry and white.

After this state of general distress has lasted for a certain time, it is succeeded by another of quite an opposite kind. The cold shivering begins to alternate with flushes of heat, which usually commence about the face and neck. By degrees the coldness ceases entirely, the skin recovers its natural colour and smoothness; the collapsed features and shrunken extremities resume their ordinary condition and bulk. But the reaction does not stop here; it goes beyond the healthy line. The face becomes red and turgid; the general surface hot, dry and pungent; the temples throb; a new kind of headache is felt; the pulse becomes full and strong, as well as rapid; the breathing is again deep, but oppressed; the urine is still scanty, but it is now high-coloured; the patient is exceedingly uncomfortable and restless. At length, another change comes over him: the skin, which from being pale and rough, had become hot and level but harsh, now recovers its natural softness; a moisture appears on the forehead and face; presently a copious and universal sweat breaks forth, with great relief to the feelings of the patient; the thirst ceases; the tongue becomes moist; the urine plentiful but turbid; the pulse regains its natural force and frequency; the pains depart; and by and by the sweating also terminates, and the patient is again as well, or nearly as well as ever.

The period that elapses between the termination of one paroxysm and the commencement of the next, is called an intermission; while the period that intervenes between the beginning of one paroxysm and the beginning of the next is called an interval. As the paroxysms are liable to vary in length, the intermissions may be very unequal, even when the intervals are the same. When the intermissions are perfect and complete, the patient resuming the appearance and sensations of health, the disorder is an intermittent fever. When the intermissions are imperfect, the patient remaining ill and feverish and uncomfortable in a less degree than during the paroxysm, then the complaint is said to be remittent fever.

Sometimes the paroxysm is incomplete: it is shorn of one or more of its stages; the heat and sweating occur without any previous shivering: or the patient shakes, but has no subsequent heat; or the sweating stage is the only one of the three that manifests itself. These fragments of a fit are often noticeable when the complaint is about to take its departure; but they may also occur at other periods of the disease. Sometimes there is no distinct stage at all; but the patient experiences frequent and irregular chills, is languid and uneasy, and depressed. This state is commonly known as the dumb ague or the dead ague.

A singular variety of Ague is recorded by Mr. Maugenet. In this case the usual order of the stages was reversed. "The patient upon each accession of the fit, was first attacked with profuse sweating, which lasted for an hour. Then the skin became dry and hot, and the face flushed, with headache, etc. This stage lasted ordinarily for five hours, when the patient began to feel cold, and eventually had distinct rigors." Quinine was as effectual in this remarkable variety, as in the regular forms of the disease.

Ague sometimes consists of a few paroxysms only, half a dozen, or four, or three, or even of one fit; or the fits may be protracted over a space of several weeks or months, or even years.

An ague may attack a person at any time; but they are much more common in spring, and in autumn, than in the other seasons of the year. The autumnal agues are the most severe and dangerous. The quotidian is most common in the spring; the quartan in the autumn; and the tertian is frequently met with both as a vernal and as an autumnal ague.

Subsequent chapters in this book give an excellent description of where and how various agues can be found, and how they are spread, and not spread. — Editor.

Bibliography

1. Other books by Joseph Blagrave:

Blagrave's Supplement or Enlargement to Mr. Nich. Culpeper's English Physitian, containing a description of the Form, Names, Place, Time and Vertues of all Medicinal Plants as grown in England. London, 1674.

Introduction to Astrology, in Three Parts. London, 1682.

2. Contemporary books of interest:

Culpeper, Nicholas: Astrological Judgement of Diseases from the Decumbiture of the Sick, 1655; and, Urinalia, 1658. Astrology Classics, Bel Air, MD, 2003

Culpeper, Nicholas: English Physitian and Complete Herbal, with Appendix, as edited by Ebenezer Sibley, 1813. *Frequently reprinted.*

Lilly, William: Christian Astrology, Modestly Treated of in Three Books, 1647. Astrology Classics, Bel Air, MD, 2004.

Saunders, Richard: The Astrological Judgement and Practice of Physick, 1677. Astrology Classics, Bel Air, MD, 2003.

3. A modern look at medieval astro-medicine:

Cornell, H.L.: Encyclopaedia of Medical Astrology. First edition 1933. Current printing: Astrology Classics, 2004.

Hofman, Oscar: Classical Medical Astrology. Wessex Astrologer, 2009

Ridder-Patrick, Jane: A Handbook of Medical Astrology, 2nd edition. CrabApple Press, 2006

4. Other books of medicinal formulas:
Brother Aloysius: A Healer's Herbal: Recipes for Medicinal Herbs and Weeds. Weiser, 1998
Smith's Family Physician, by William Henry Smith. John Lovell, 1873.

5. A little bit on witchcraft:
Fortune, Diane: Psychic Self-Defense. Weiser, 2001.

6. On "Sympathetic healing":
Choa Kok Sui: Advanced Pranic Healing. Weiser, 1995.
Choa Kok Sui: Miracles Through Pranic Healing. Institute for Inner Studies, Makati City, Philippines, 1999.
Choa Kok Sui: Pranic Psychotherapy. Weiser, 1993.

Index

45 degrees, 34
Abortion, to hinder, 83
Aches, coming of cold, 83
Aches, coming of heat, 83
Aches, ulcers, wounds, burnings or scaldings, 77
Acute diseases, 27
Acute griefs, xxxvii, 33, 36
Afflicted, 27
Afflicted under Sun and Mercury, 110
Afterbirth and secundine to expel, 83
Agrippa, Cornelius, xxxv, 24
Agues, xxxvii, xxxviii, xxxix, 75, 169-171, 176, 177, 180
Agues, cure, 83, 173-178
Alcohol, xv, xvi
Aldermaston, near Reading, 115
Almanacks, 1658, 1659, xxxvi, xxxviii
Antipathetical, 49, 75, 77, 122, 126, 130, 143-4, 145, 180, 182
Antipathy, xxxiii, xxxiv, xxxvi, xxxviii, xl, 113, 115, 128, 180, 182
Apoplexies, 35
Apoplexies, to cure, 84
Apostles, xxxvii, 124
Apostumes, to cure, 84
Appetite, to procure, 84
Aquarius body, ailments, 58
Aries body, ailments, 56
Ascella Publishing, xvii, xviii, xix, xx
Ascendant, observations, 50
Ascendant, sixth and twelfth houses, 28
Ascendant, sixth house, lords afflicted, 46
Ascendant, true, 51
Ascendant, vary, v, 37, 42, 52, 158
Ascendant, wrong, 51
Aspect, friendly, 55
Astral, xv, xvi
Atakes, 120. *See also* Evils, Takes
Atrophy or wasting limbs, to cure, 147
Auras, viii
Azimene degrees, 54, 195
Back and reins, to strengthen, 84

Barrenness, to help, 84
Baths, 124, 128, 143
Baths and fomentations, 77
Baths and sweats, 80
Bear cream, 138
Bedlam, 182
Bedridden, 122
Belching, to repress, 84
Belly, to bind, 85
Belly, to loosen, 85
Bellyache, 84
Berm, 72
Bible, astrology, 152
Bladder, to cleanse, 85
Blagrave's Supplement or Enlargement to Nich. Culpeper, xix
Bleeding, to stay, 85
Blind, 18
Blood, xiii, xvi, xxxiv
Blood over heated, 49
Blood, let, 31, 49, 80, 123, 127, 135, 142, 149, 176, 177, 178, 180, 181
Blood, let, choleric, 81
Blood, let, elder people, 81
Blood, let, melancholy, 81
Blood, let, middle age, 81
Blood, let, old people, 81
Blood, let, phlegmatic, 81
Blood, let, sanguine, 81
Blood, let, young, 81
Blood, to cleanse, 85
Bloody brandy, xiv. *See also* Spirit of Wine
Body shape, 42
Boil close covered, 71
Boiling in milk, 74
Bole Armeniac, 136
Bound, bound in body, 74, 116, 182
Boy bewitched, 132
Breast and stomach, to cleanse, 85
Breath, stinking, to help, 85
Broken bones, to help knit, 86
Brown's daughter, cured, 110

Burgundy pitch, 76
Burnings and scaldings, to cure, 86
Burstings or ruptures, to cure, 86
Cancer body, ailments, 57
Capricorn body, ailments, 58
Carbuncles, to cure, 86
Cast out spirits, devils, x, xi
Catalogue of herbs, to cure, 82-109
Cataplasms, ix, 75, 113, 115, 116, 127, 176, 177
Catarrhs or thin rheums, to stay, 86
Celandine-water, 119
Chakra, crown, xi
Chakras, viii, xi
Chakras, minor, ix
Charm, 134
Child birth, to help, 86
Choler, 180
Choler and Phlegm, to purge, 86
Choleric, xxxvii, 111
Choleric or sanguine, xxxvi
Choleric people, 111
Cholic of wind, to ease, 87
Christian Astrology, vi
Chronic, 28, 31
Chronic diseases, 27
Chronic griefs, 37
Cliches of the arms, 116
Cold and dry, xxxvi, 7, 8, 10, 11, 113
Cold and moist, 8, 9, 11, 49, 113
Cold dryness, 116
Cold infirmities, 80
Colds, coughs and hoarseness, to cure, 87
Collins, a baker, his daughter, 112
Combustion, free of, 32
Complexion, xl
Compliance, xxxix
Conjunction, platic, 50
Consumptions, dropsies, agues, gouts, 54
Consumptions, to cure, 87
Contrary nature, 77-8
Convulsion fits, 112, 113-4
Convulsions, 35, 110
Convulsions, apoplexies, palpitations, 75
Convulsions, to cure, 87
Cooling and cleansing, 49
Cooling remedies, xl
Costive, bound, 74, 181
Course, monthly, 182
Courses of women, to provoke, 87
Courses of women, to stop, 88
Cramps, to ease, 88

Credits, xxi
Crisis, first, 30
Critical figure, 30, 33
Critical figure of 16 parts, 36
Critical, intercidental, judicial, 28, 29, 30
Crucial circle of 16 equal parts, 30
Cure at Berkshire, 115
Cure, unsatisfied, xxxvi
Cures, two at Oxon, 110
Daily fits, 126
Dandelion, 14
Days of week, rulerships, v
Dead palsy, xxxix, 115, 122
Deafness, to cure, 88
Death or recovery, 35
Death, signs, 55
Death, testimonies, 32
Decoctions, xxxv, 73 74, 119, 126, 128, 180
Decoctions and diet-drinks, 71
Decoctions, syrups or cordials, 49
Decumbiture, xii, xxxvii, 37, 42, 51
Decumbiture, another judgement, 35
Decumbiture, figure for the time of, 43
Decumbiture, imaginary, 32
Decumbiture, judgement, 47
Decumbiture, time of, 50
Degrees first and second, 8
Degrees third and fourth, 7, 8, 9
Degrees, first, second, third, fourth, 7
Devils, casting forth, 159-166
Diet drinks, way to make, 71
Diet-drink three times a day 71
Diet-drinks, xxxiv, 113, 116, 119, 122, 124, 126, 127, 131, 135, 176, 177, 180, 182
Digestion and concoction, to help, 88
Diseases, how to discover, 27
Distemper of heart and brain, 110
Distemper, discover, 51
Distemper, feverish, 49
Distemper, present, 48
Dogs mad, their bitings to cure, 88
Dragon's head, 33
Dropsical humors, 128
Dropsy, to cure, 89
Drugs, xxxiii, xxxiv
Drug-Doctors, 110
dryness or moisture, 10
Dumb spirit, casting out, 167-9
Dung, excrement, x, 145
Earrings, ix

Index

Ears, pain and noise, to help, 89
Eclipse of Sun or Moon, 56
Edward, King, 118
Elemental qualities, xl, 7, 9, 10, 13, 15, 113
Elemental qualities, first, xxxvii, 14
Ephemeris, 40
Ephemeris for 1658, 151
Ephemeris, use, 41
Erecting a figure, xxxvii
Etheric, xv, xvi
Evil upon the maid, 112
Evil, ear and right side of head, 119
Evils, xxxvii, 113
Evils or takes, 124, 143
External healing, part 1, vii
Externalization of diseases, x
Extractions, xxxv
Eyes, inflamed, red or bloodshot, to cure, 89
Eyesight, to quicken, 89
Falling sickness, 89, 110
Fascination, 132
Fascination, witchcraft or sorcery, 174
Fast, 78
Fees, xvii
Fevers, burning, to cure, 90
Fevers, convulsions, apoplexies, risings in the throat, pestilential infirmities, 54
Fevers, pestilential, to cure, 90
Fevers, to cure, 90
Figure of 12 houses, 37
Figure of 12 houses, how to give judgement, 45
Figure of twelve houses, 27
First and eighth hours, 17
First, fourth, sixth, eighth, twelfth houses, 51
Fit, strong, 51
Fits, 135
Flegm, to purge, 90
Flowers of women, 90
Flux of the belly and humours, to stop, 90
Flux or lask, 48
Flux, bloody, to stay, 90
Fluxes, rheums and laxes, 80
Fortunes, influential virtue, 16
French pox, to cure, 91
Fugitives, 157
Fumes, 75, 180
Fundament, falling, to remedy, 91
Gall, to open, 91

Gathering herbs and plants, controversy, 14
Gemini, 52
Gemini body, ailments, 57
Glisters, 49, 74, 80, 116, 128, 181, 182
God, duty towards, 125
Gold, vii, 111, 113, 118, 130
Gold crosses, viii
Gold rings, viii, ix
Good smell and taste, 11
Good to comfort the vertue, the Moon in, 81
Google Books, xviii
Gout, hot or cold, to cure, 147
Gout, to cure, 92
Greensickness, to cure, 91
Gregorian calendar, iii
Grief, cold, xxxix
Grief, discover, 48
Grief, mortal, 34
Grief, what it is, 47
Griefs, fixed stars, 56
Griefs, obscure, 46
Guts stopped, to cure, 92
Hand, severed, xvi
Hand-wrists, 113, 116, 127, 176, 177. *See also* Wrists.
Harp (Wega) fixed star, 48
Harvesting organs, xvi
Hazel tree, 147
Head and brain disaffected, 75
Head giddiness and swimmings, to cure, 92
Head, to purge, 92
Headache, to cure, 92
Headache, to draw to the feet, 92
Hearing loss, to cure, 93
Heart vein, 135
Heart, pains at, 35
Heart, to fortify against infection, 92
Hearts, fainting or palpitations, to cure, 93
Heat, xxxix
Heat and dryness, 15
Heat or cold, 9, 10, 13
Hemorrhoids or piles, to cure, 93
Herbs and planets, how to gather, 17
Herbs and plants, catalog, 1-6
Herbs and plants, general rules, 7
Herbs heating and binding, 74
Herbs, gathering, 13
Hernia or rupture, to cure, 148

Hiccups, to stay, 93
Hoarseness and loss of voice, to help, 93
Horary questions, 150
Hot and dry, 8, 9, 10, 49, 113
Hot and moist, xxxvi, 8, 113
Hot baths, 112
Hot diseases, 80
Hot or cold, 14
Hot or cold swellings, 77
Hours, January, 18
Hours, February, 18
Hours, March, 19
Hours, April, 19
Hours, May, 20
Hours, June, 20
Hours, July, 21
Hours, August, 21
Hours, September, 22
Hours, October, 22
Hours, November, 23
Hours, December, 23
How to erect a scheme or figure, 41
Humors, gross, to expel, 93
Iliac passion, to cure, 92
Ill of long continuance, 124
Image, 121, 126, 137
Image or model, 120, 124, 143
Infirmities, natural, 49
Inflammations, to assuage, 94
Infused a spirit, 131
Inscriptions, xvi
Intercidental time, first, 34
Intercidental, judicial, 36
Itches, to cure, 94
Jaundies, black, 32
Jaundies, yellow, 109
Jaundies, yellow, to cure, 94
Jelly of calves legs, 113
Jesus Christ, 132
Jewelry, ix
Joints, pained, 94
Judicial time, 34
Jugular, ix
Julian calendar, iii
Jupiter herbs, 1-2
Jupiter, body, ailments, 59
Jupiter, hot and moist, 111
Jupiter, Venus or the Sun, 46
Kernals and knots in the flesh, to cure, 94
Kernals, white, 111, 117, 131
Kidneys, to cleanse, 95
King's Evil, 111, 117, 121, 131

Kings Evil, to cure, 95
Kinsman, friend or acquaintance, during absence, 149
Lasks or looseness, to stay, 95
Latitude, iii
Legality of practice, xvii, xxxvi, xxxvii, xxxviii, 151
Legend of planets, xxi
Legend of signs, xxi
Leo body, ailments, 57
Leo, lord, falling sick, 51
Leprosy, to cure, 95
Lethargy or drowsy evil, to cure, 96
Libra body, ailments, 58
License, 115
Life, testimonies, 33
Lilly, William, vi, xii, xiii
Limbeck still, 72
Liquorice stick, 73
Live or die, 35, 47
Liver obstructed, to open and purge, 96
Lohocks and Lambatives, to make, 73
London Dispensary, 73, 79
Lord of ascendant combust, 55
Lord of the ascendant, 54, 55
Lord of the ascendant in an earthy sign, 80
Lord of the hour, 14
Lord of the sixth, 46
Lord of the twelfth, 46, 126 132
Lungs, to open and cleanse, 96
Madness, with way of cure, 179-183
Magnet of one's own body, 145
Man's blood, 136
Man's grease, xvi, 136
Mars herbs, 2-3
Mars, body, ailments, 60
Mars, choler, 78
Mastiff dog, 133
Melancholy, xxxvii, 111, 180
Melancholy blood, 32
Melancholy cold planets, 111
Melancholy, to repress and purge, 96
Mercury herbs, 5-6
Mercury, body, ailments, 60
Mercury, cold and dry, 111
Milk, to cause in women's breast, 97
Milk, to dry up in women's breast, 97
Mind, to know at a distance, 149
Mirth, to cause, 96
Moisture, xxxix
Moon afflicted, 46, 49

Index

Moon afflicted in the fourth or eighth, 55
Moon and Mercury principally concerned, 112
Moon applying to combustion, 56
Moon herbs, 6
Moon in acute griefs, afflicted, 55
Moon in Aquarius of Mars afflicted, 35, 65
Moon in Aquarius of Saturn or Mercury oppressed, 70
Moon in Aries of Mars afflicted, 62
Moon in Aries of Saturn or Mercury oppressed, 66
Moon in aspect with Mars or Saturn, vi
Moon in Cancer of Mars afflicted, 63
Moon in Cancer of Saturn or Mercury oppressed, 67
Moon in Capricorn of Mars afflicted, 65
Moon in Capricorn of Saturn or Mercury oppressed, 69
Moon in common sign, 48
Moon in Gemini of Mars afflicted, 63
Moon in Gemini of Saturn or Mercury oppressed, 67
Moon in Leo of Mars afflicted, 63
Moon in Leo of Saturn oppressed, 32
Moon in Leo of Saturn or Mercury oppressed, 68
Moon in Libra of Mars afflicted, 64
Moon in Libra of Saturn or Mercury oppressed, 68
Moon in Pisces of Mars afflicted, 66
Moon in Pisces of Saturn or Mercury oppressed, 70
Moon in Sagittarius of Mars afflicted, 65
Moon in Sagittarius of Mars oppressed, 29
Moon in Sagittarius of Saturn or Mercury oppressed, 69
Moon in Scorpio of Mars afflicted, 64
Moon in Scorpio of Saturn or Mercury oppressed, 69
Moon in Taurus of Mars afflicted, 62
Moon in Taurus of Saturn or Mercury oppressed, 67
Moon in Virgo of Mars afflicted, vi, 64
Moon in Virgo of Saturn or Mercury oppressed, 68
Moon in watery signs, 77, 78
Moon increasing in light, 55
Moon meets opposition of Mars, 36
Moon, applying to the lord of the ascendant, 56
Moon, body, ailments, 61
Moon, increasing in light, 32
Moon, judgement by, 45
Mortal time, 30
Moss of a dead man's skull, xvi, 136
Mother fits, 35
Mother fits, suffocation or risings, to cure, 96
Motion, swift, 54
Mummy, 136
Multiple personality disorder, xi
Nature, contrary, 144
Nerves, 117
Nerves and arteries oppressed, 110
New Style, iii
Nose bleeding, to stop, 97
Number, xxxv
Numbers, Jupiter, 24
Numbers, lesser and greater, 120
Numbers, Mars, 25
Numbers, Mercury, 26
Numbers, Moon, 26
Numbers, Saturn, 24
Numbers, Sol, 25
Numbers, Venus, 25
Numbness, to remove, 97
Oak, 147
Obstructions, to remove, 97
Oil of lindseed, 136
Oil of roses, 136
Oil of young puppies, 113
Oil to anoint the brain, 119
Oils, 113, 115, 116
Ointment, subtle 136
Ointments, 74, 76, 77, 119, 122, 124, 127, 128, 131, 137, 143, 180, 182
Old Style, iii
Open and cleanse, 10
Opening plants, 98
Opposition, partile, 32
Opposition, platic, 32
Orbs, 15
Pagination, xviii, xix, xx
Pain and pricking at the heart, 123
Palms, ix
Palpitations, vii
Palsy, to cure, 98
Patient body bound, 78
Patient troubled with wind, 71
Patient, age, xxxvi
Patient, complexion, xxxvi

Patient, old, xxxix
Patient, visit, 42, 50
Peracute, 31
Peracute griefs, 34
Peregrine, 33
Perperacute mortal sickness, 31
Perperacute sickness, 34
Perpetual almanac, iii
Phlegmatic, xxxvii, 180
Piles, to cure, 98
Pills, 116
Pills, to make and use, 73
Pisces body, ailments, 59
Plague, 34
Plague or pestilence, to cure or prevent, 98
Plague-sore, to cure, 148
Planet, fortunate, 36
Planetary hour, wrong, xxxiv
Planetary hours, iv, xxxiii, xxxv, 13, 17, 74, 111, 119,
Planetary hours, nighttime, iv
Planetary hours, rulerships, iv
Planets in figures, 44
Planets, both influence, 15
Planets, characters, 38
Planets, five aspects, 38
Planets, houses, 39
Plants and herbs, iii
Plants and herbs, spirits to extract, 72
Plants, blossoms, 10
Pleurisy, to cure, 98
Poison, resist, xxxvi
Poisonous matter prepared, 138
Posset drink, 177
Pranic Healing, x
Pray and preach against, 114
Prayer, xiii, xiv
Prayer to God, 125
Prayers, morning, 125
Prayers, neglect of, 132
Pre-Copernican world, 194
Prick about the heart, 126
Pricked in the head, 123
Psychic, xvi
Ptisick, to cure, 99
Pulvus Sanctus, 79
Purgations, 77, 181
Purge, xxxiv
Purge blood, 78 79
Purge choler, 79
Purge flegm, 78

Purge flegm and water, 79
Purge melancholy, 78, 79
Purge the head, 79
Purge, strong, 78
Purging and loosening, 182
Purging the body, 78
Purging the body of ill humors, 99
Purples, to cure, 99
Quartan ague, 172-3
Quartans, xxxviii
Quartile aspect, 33
Quinsey, to cure, 99
Quotidian fits, 176
Quotidian agues, 170
Raw-fresh meat, 119
Reconcile rules, 14
Recovery, rules, 54
Recovery, signs of, 47
Recovery, time, 48
Recovery, way of, 49
Reins, to cleanse, 99
Relapses, 135
Rest, to procure, 100
Retrograde, 54, 154
Retrograde planets, 77, 80
Rheums, to stay, 100
Rickets, 100
Ringworms, 100
Rising in the throat by way of flegm, 110
Roman-vitriol, 119, 133
Roses, herbs or flowers, 72
Ruby, 131
Running of the reins, to cure, 99
Ruptures, 100
Sagittarius body, ailments, 58
Saint Anthony's Fire, 84
Sal-Gem, 74, 78
Sallet oil, 74
Sanguine, xxxvii, 180
Saturn afflicting planet, 115
Saturn herbs, 1
Saturn not an enemy, 50
Saturn, body, ailments, 59
Saturn, Mars, Mercury or the Sun, 46
Scabs and scurfs, to heal, 100
Scald head, to cure, 100
Scaldings, to cure, 100
Sciatica or hip gout, to cure, 100
Scorpio body, ailments, 58
Scurvy, to cure, 104
Self-defense, xiii
Semi-semi-quartile aspect, 34

Semination or transplantation, 146
Separating and applying, 15
Serpents stinging, or venomous bitings, to cure, 101
Shingles, to cure, 104
Shrank up both legs, 112
Sick depart, 31
Sick first takes to bed, 28
Sick man's glass, 39
Sick person will die, 36
Sick recovers, 33
Sick, personate, 42, 50
Sick, recovered, 47
Sick, significator, changing signs, 53
Sickness long and short, brief rules, 53
Significator, principal, xxxv
Signs, body shape, 56
Signs, characters, 38
Signs, common, weeks, 53
Signs, fixed, months, 53
Signs, latter degrees, 54
Signs, moveable, days, 53
Sinews shrinking, to help, 103
Sinews, to strengthen, 103
Siphon, siphoning, x, xiii
Sixth cusp, fixed sign, 53
Sixth house, 50
Sixth house, lord, 49
Sleep, to procure, 104
Solary herbs, xxxvi, xl, 119, 120, 144
Solary herbs, bath, 119
Solary herbs, three, vii, 111, 113, 118, 130
Solary herbs, wear a select number, 144
Solary plants, to wear, 176
Sorcery, xii, 126, 127, 143
Sorcery or witchcraft, 176, 182
Sorcery, witchcraft, 141
Sounding fits, 123
Source text, xvii
Spelling, xx
Spirit of wine, xv, 72, 149. *See also* Bloody brandy
Spitting of blood, to stay, 103
Spleens, diseases, obstructions and inward swellings, to cure, 101
Spots, freckles and pimples, to clear, 103
Square, partile, 35
Square, platic, 28, 49
Stature, large, fat, full and fleshy, 51
Stibium, 177
Stitches or side pains, to ease, 102

Stomach bad, to help cleanse and strengthen, 101
Stone, 102
Stone and gravel, to expel, 102
Stone in the kidneys and reins, to expel, 102
Stool, 78
Strangury or pissing stopped, to help, 103
Struck dumb, 129
Suffumigations, 75, 116, 131, 180
Sun herbs, 3-4
Sun in chronic, afflicted, 55
Sun on Sundays, 17
Sun, body, ailments, 60
Sunrise, first half hour, iv
Suppository, 74, 78, 116, 181
Surfeiting, 49
Surfeits, to cure, 104
Swan's bill (Albireo) fixed star, 48
Sweats, 128
Sweet smell, 15
Swelling, sore, schirrous tumor, warts, to cure, 146, 147
Swelling, white, 119, 121
Swellings, 103
Swellings in the eyes, 111
Swellings in the throat, 111
Swooning fits, 35
Swoonings and faintings, to cure, 103
Swounding fits, 32
Sympathetic, 9, 119
Sympathetic cures, x
Sympathetic powder, to apply, 134
Sympathetical powder, x, 132, 178, 180
Sympathy, xiii, xxxii, xxxiv, xxxv, xxxvi, xxxviii, xxxix, 126, 137, 139, 143
Sympathy and antipathy, 12
Sympathy or antipathy, 146
Syrups, to make, 72
Table of essential dignities, 195
Takes, 121
Taurus body, ailments, 56
Terms, 104
Tertian ague, 171-2
Tetters, to heal, 104
Thefts and strays amongst cattle, 154
Thief, described, 156
Thorn, pin or needle, 120
Throat-almonds, to help, 104
Throat-soreness and diseases, to help, 105
Throats inflammations to assuage, 105
Throats kernels and swellings, to waste,

105
Tilehurst, 115
Time of falling ill, 41
Time of recovery, 30
Time of recovery, expected, 31
Time, mortal, 36
Toothache, 137
Toothache, to help, 105
Tragacanth, gum, 73
Transplant, 145
Twelfth house, 46, 47
Two scholars, 114
Typesetting, xx
Ulcers, hollow, and fistulas, to cleanse, 106
Ulcers and sores, to heal, 105
Ulcers in the privy parts, to cure, 106
Ulcers or sores running and spreading, to cure, 106
Ulcers, hollow to fill with flesh, 106
Unguent, or wonderful ointment for wounds, 136
Unlawful cure, 114
Urine, xiii, xxxiv, xxxvii, 110, 137, 141, 142
Urine in horary, 158
Urine, amber color, 158
Urine, brought, 50
Urine, cleanse the passages, 10
Urine, first brought, 42
Urine, flinty and thick, 159
Urine, gravel or red sand, 159
Urine, green or black, 159
Urine, high coloured and red, 158
Urine, light sandy color, 159
Urine, receipt, 51
Urine, sad brown colour, 159
Urine, to provoke, 106
Urine, white or palish, 158
Usurer, 114
Venomous beasts, or vipers biting, to cure, 107
Venus herbs, 4-5
Venus turpentine, 76
Venus, body, ailments, 60
Verjuice posset, 122
Vertigo, 107
Via combusta, 29 32 47
Virgo body, ailments, 57
Vomit, xxxiv, 177
Vomiting, to repress, 107
Vomits, 80

Voodoo, xii
Vulva fallen, to help, 107
Water gruel or broth, 72
Water-gruel, 116, 127, 131
Water-gruel or thin broth, 78
Weak and peregrine, 115
Wear about the neck, 130
Whites or reds, to stay, 108
Wickens, Peter, 115
Willow-tree, 147
Wind, to expel, 108
Witch, 123, 124, 129, 139, 175
Witch's significator, 142
Witch, afflict, 122, 126, 130, 140, 141, 176
Witch, black, 124, 140
Witch, vital spirit, 139
Witch, white, 124, 140
Witchcraft, xi, xii, xiii, xvi, xvii, 27, 37, 47, 120, 121, 125, 126, 131, 132
Witchcraft and sorcery, 52, 121, 122, 123, 137
Witchcraft and sorcery, cure, 140
Witchcraft or sorcery, 46, 143, 170, 179
Witchcraft, sorcery, 138
Witches, suspected, 125
Womb, to open and cleanse, 108
Women's courses, 10
Worms, to kill, 108
Wounds, green, to help, 109
Wounds, inflammations to assuage, 109
Wounds, to heal, 109
Wrists, ix. *See also* Hand-wrists.
Writing which the patient wears, 178. *See also* Inscriptions.
Youth and age, xxxvii

Better books make better astrologers.
Here are some of our other titles:

AstroAmerica's Daily Ephemeris, 2010-2020
AstroAmerica's Daily Ephemeris, 2000-2020
  - all for Midnight. Compiled & formatted by David R. Roell

Al Biruni
The Book of Instructions in the Elements of the Art of Astrology, *1029 AD, translated by R. Ramsay Wright*

Derek Appleby
Horary Astrology: The Art of Astrological Divination

E. H. Bailey
The Prenatal Epoch

C.E.O. Carter
An Encyclopaedia of Psychological Astrology
The Principles of Astrology, *Intermediate no. 1*
Some Principles of Horoscopic Delineation, *Intermediate no. 2*

Charubel & Sepharial
Degrees of the Zodiac Symbolized, *1898*

Nicholas Culpeper
Astrological Judgement of Diseases from the Decumbiture of the Sick, *1655, and,* **Urinalia**, *1658*

Dorotheus of Sidon
Carmen Astrologicum, *c. 50 AD, translated by David Pingree*

Nicholas deVore
Encyclopedia of Astrology

Firmicus Maternus
Ancient Astrology Theory & Practice: Matheseos Libri VIII, *c. 350 AD, translated by Jean Rhys Bram*

William Lilly
Christian Astrology, books 1 & 2, *1647*
  The Introduction to Astrology, Resolution of all manner of questions.
Christian Astrology, book 3, *1647*
  Easie and plaine method teaching how to judge upon nativities.

Alan Leo
The Progressed Horoscope, *1905*

Jean-Baptiste Morin
The Cabal of the Twelve Houses Astrological, *translated by George Wharton, edited by D.R. Roell*

Claudius Ptolemy
Tetrabiblos, *c. 140 AD, translated by J.M. Ashmand*
The great book, in the classic translation.

Vivian Robson
Astrology and Sex
Electional Astrology
Fixed Stars & Constellations in Astrology

Richard Saunders
The Astrological Judgement and Practice of Physick, *1677*
By the Richard who inspired Ben Franklin's famous Almanac.

Sepharial
Primary Directions, a definitive study
A complete, detailed guide.

Sepharial On Money. *For the first time in one volume, complete texts:*
- **Law of Values**
- **Silver Key**
- **Arcana, or Stock and Share Key** — *first time in print!*

James Wilson, Esq.
Dictionary of Astrology
From 1820. Quirky, opinionated, a fascinating read.

H.S. Green, Raphael & C.E.O. Carter
Mundane Astrology: *3 Books, complete in one volume.*
A comprehensive guide to political astrology

If not available from your local bookseller, order directly from:
The Astrology Center of America
207 Victory Lane
Bel Air, MD 21014

on the web at:
http://www.astroamerica.com